Trigeminal neuralgia: a complete guide book.

Trigeminal neuralgia: causes, symptoms, treatments, surgery, pain relief, risk factors and prevention.

By
Robert Rymore

Co-Author:
Dr. Tulsi Dabhi
Alternative Therapist, Professor of Medicine, Medical writer

Table of Contents

Table of Contents

Preface

In recent years, the medical profession has evolved more than it has ever evolved in the last few decades. With advancement in medical science and technology, the physicians who were earlier known to be holistic healers, have become victims of machinery and time, and have gradually become very mechanical in treating their patients. They have learnt to put much thought into the treatment of the patient rather than using their heart to cure. Trigeminal neuralgia is one of the most harrowing illnesses. It can only be treated effectively when every physician takes a holistic approach in treating the patient along with complementing various lifestyle changes, alternative therapies, psychological support and appropriate medico-surgical treatment. In this book we have tried to incorporate each and every minute detail related to the Trigeminal neuralgia. This book is dedicated to all trigeminal neuralgia patients, their family members and the physicians in order to take the first step towards the comprehensive cure for the trigeminal neuralgia.

Acknowledgement

It is my proud privilege to express my deepest regards to all my teachers for giving me a sound base of fundamental principles of medicine.

I am grateful to all my patients, whose suffering was my inspiration for writing this book in order to resolve each and every problem.

Special thanks to my husband and my children who always motivated me to do something different and all the love and positivity they give me. Without their support it won't be possible to give my 100% to this book.

Thank you all.

Chapter 1: Trigeminal Neuralgia, What is it all about?

Any disorder of the nervous system is one of the most common debilitating conditions that can affect an individual. One of the reasons that these conditions have more lasting and sometimes irreversible effects is due to the damage occurred to the nervous tissues, rendering it unable to carry out its normal functions. Conditions affecting the nervous systems have effects in almost all parts of the body, either in local or systemic effect. In addition to this, most of these conditions have no apparent causes, or risk factors related to their existence are widely unknown, so treatment is often hard or challenging not only for the individuals, but also for the doctors caring for them. Moreover, most of the conditions involving the nervous system cause pain, rendering the person unable to carry out his day to day activities with ease and increasing his risks to develop psychosocial problems such as feelings of isolation and depression.

Among these conditions of the nervous system that affects individuals globally, trigeminal neuralgia is one of the most common. It is mostly misdiagnosed as being a sign of hypochondriasis, or diagnosed lately due to the non-specific symptoms. It has been tagged as the *suicide disease*, since the intense and severe pain felt by individuals suffering from it is debilitating, even extending for a longer period of time. This is what leads the trigeminal neuralgia patients to contemplate committing suicide to end their suffering with intense pain caused by trigeminal neuralgia.

This book is all about trigeminal neuralgia and is divided into several chapters to thoroughly discuss and present information to the non-medical individuals. The first chapter contains the background into the problem of trigeminal neuralgia. It also covers the basic anatomy and physiology of the trigeminal nerve and its associated branches, the identified subtypes of trigeminal neuralgia, most common symptoms, its causes and how it can affect the life of the individual suffering from it. Chapter two is about the history of trigeminal neuralgia. It discusses how the condition that we now know has evolved and changed in the perception of doctors and individuals and when it was first noted to exist. This chapter also includes snippets of information about some of the most famous personalities who have suffered from trigeminal neuralgia.

The third chapter of this book talks about risk factors on the development of trigeminal neuralgia, categorizing them as modifiable and non-modifiable risk factors. The next chapter, chapter four is all about how to arrive at the diagnosis of trigeminal neuralgia and the assessment tests that can be performed on the individual to rule out or confirm its presence. Chapter five is all about treatment options available to those who are suffering from the condition. It talks about invasive and non-invasive therapies, medications and even how alternative and traditional medicine may help treat the condition and provide optimal pain relief. The chapter also talks about these treatments objectively, presenting both the advantages and disadvantages of each treatment regimen. The sixth chapter talks about the relationship between dental problems and procedures and the diagnosis of trigeminal neuralgia. It gives light to how the condition is often misdiagnosed as a dental problem and how dental procedures can affect it positively and negatively.

The seventh chapter discusses the different ways of coping with the problem once it is diagnosed and how to maintain independence and pain-free episodes. The next chapter, chapter 8 details ways on how to avoid developing the problem and decreasing a person's risk factor for suffering from this debilitating facial pain. And finally, chapter 9 summarizes all the points made in this book, and provides a conclusion.

1) Overview of the Condition

The Anatomy and Physiology of the Trigeminal Nerve

The trigeminal nerve is one of the 12 cranial nerves that originates from the brain and controls most sensory and motor functions along the areas traversed by its pathways. It is the fifth of the 12 cranial nerves and functions both as a sensory and motor nerve. This means that apart from being responsible to facilitate perception and transmission of sensory impulses, it also plays an important role in controlling certain movements of the face. The sensory portions of this nerve and its branches are formed by the nerves found mainly in the maxillary, mandibular and ophthalmic areas of the face. These are responsible for transmission of stimuli introduced upon the face, in some portions of the mouth and along the teeth and gum line to the brain to be interpreted as sensations. The ophthalmic branch is responsible for the interpretation of sensation in the eyes, along the sinuses and the skin on the forehead and the nose. The maxillary branch's area of functioning is the lower eyelids, along the sides of the nose and the upper lip. The mandibular branch affects sensory perception along the jaw line, the area behind the ears, lower side of the face and two thirds of the tongue. These nerve fibers can be traced in their origins at the trigeminal ganglion and also in the brain stem where the trigeminal nucleus is found. The motor function of the trigeminal nerve, however, originates from the brain stem and has the responsibility of governing the muscles of the cheek and jaw area, helping in carrying out the process of mastication, or chewing.

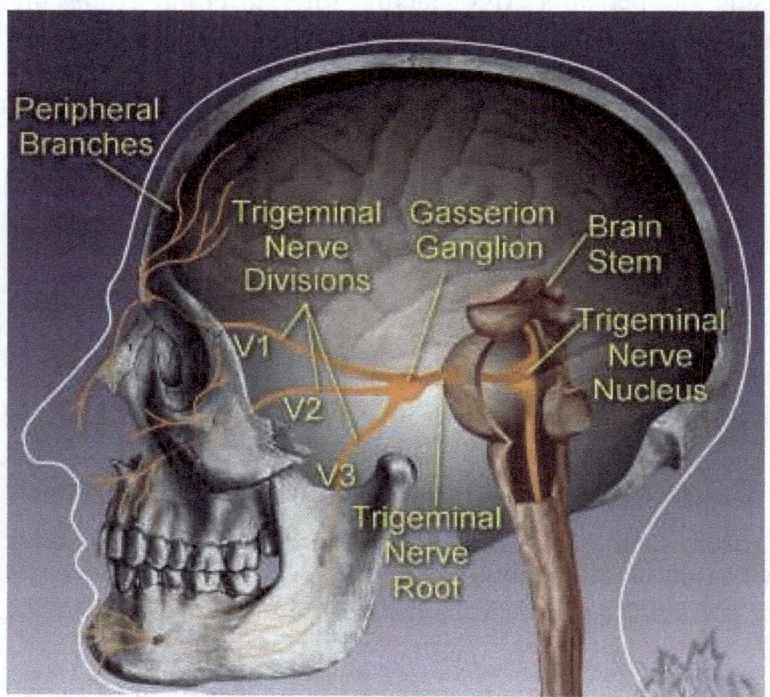

Source: Center for Cranial Nerve Disorders
http://www.umanitoba.ca

The Trigeminal Nerve

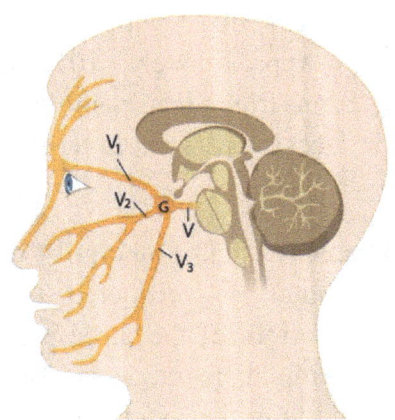

2) Trigeminal Neuralgia and its Definition

Trigeminal neuralgia is a disorder of the nervous system that is usually associated with instances where the affected individual experiences intense pain in specific areas of the face where the trigeminal nerve traverses. It is known as other names such as occipital neuralgia, tic doulourex, and neuralgia del trigemino in Spanish-speaking individuals.

The trigeminal nerve, or CN V (Cranial Nerve 5), is a cranial nerve that has a sensory function, meaning its main purpose is to distinguish sensations that are introduced along the area of its distribution. It is a paired cranial nerve having branches in the ophthalmic (or the area near the eyes), maxillary and mandibular (areas close to and along the jaw line). These areas are usually marked with the legend V_1, V_2, and V_3 respectively in most literature sources. These nerve areas are usually affected, either singly or collectively. However, the most commonly affected among these three branches is the middle or the maxillary branch and the mandibular branch. These areas include the individual suffering from pain in areas of the face such as the ears, the eyes, nose, along the jaw or gum line, cheeks, lips, scalp, forehead and sometimes even in the teeth. Approximately 10% of all individuals who are suffering from trigeminal neuralgia have affection of both sides of their faces, and what is termed as a bilateral condition.

The condition is also known in names such as Fothergill's disease or prosopalgia. Trigeminal neuralgia is considered to be a neuropathic disorder, meaning the origin of the disease itself is nervous in nature. Moreover, trigeminal neuralgia is also often associated with *tic doloreux*, a condition that is characterized by muscular spasms on one side of the face (or hemifacial spasms). This condition is usually described as one of the most painful conditions that can ever affect an individual, and one of those that brings about psychosocial problems to its victim.

Trigeminal neuralgia affects people all over the world, with an estimated prevalence of 1 in every 15,000 or 20,000 of population. This figure, however, may be lower than the actual number of people affected with it since there is a chance that it may have been unreported or misdiagnosed in many instances. The condition may also occur in all ages, although most of those afflicted with it report an onset of symptoms at the age of 50. For some unknown reason, trigeminal neuralgia is more commonly seen in females than in males.

3) Subtypes of Trigeminal Neuralgia

At present, there are seven subtypes of trigeminal neuralgia that are recognized in the medical world. These subtypes are usually named after an associated condition. The seven subtypes are known as: typical type trigeminal neuralgia, atypical type (ATN), pre-TN subtype, secondary type trigeminal neuralgia, post-traumatic trigeminal neuralgia (usually known as trigeminal neuropathy), multiple sclerosis related trigeminal neuralgia and failed type neuralgia.

Typical Trigeminal Neuralgia

The most commonly occurring among these seven subtypes is the typical trigeminal neuralgia. It is also referred to as *tic doloreux* in most literatures. Typical trigeminal neuralgia has also been termed as Essential, Idiopathic and Classical trigeminal neuralgia in the past. The pain that is associated with typical neuralgia is usually described as being intense, and likened to an electric shock. It can also be characterized as stabbing in some cases. The main problem in this type of neuralgia is that there is a marked compression of the blood vessels supplying the root of the trigeminal nerve, which happens to the point where it enters the brainstem. This compression of the smaller blood vessels and nerves at the trigeminal areas are usually caused by bigger problems in the arteries or veins near the trigeminal nerve. This is an alteration in the anatomy and physiology in that specific area, since people who are not affected with trigeminal neuralgia; should have no sign of compression of the nerves and the vessels in the root portion of the trigeminal nerve.

Normally, there are pulsations present in the trigeminal nerve that are brought about by the action of the blood along the vessel walls but these pulsations are not strong enough to cause visible damages. These are also not enough to cause alterations in the functioning of the nerves as well. The problem lies therefore in the pulsations that occur repeatedly and are sustained over a long period of time, causing changes in the functioning of the nerves and brings about an alteration to the signal delivery along the nucleus of the trigeminal nerve. When this condition persists over an extended period of time, the nucleus of the trigeminal nerve becomes hyperactive, leading to transmission of pain impulses that are interpreted as trigeminal nerve pain.

Atypical Trigeminal Neuralgia

Another subtype is the Type 2 Trigeminal Neuralgia, or what is being considered as the atypical trigeminal neuralgia, medically referred as ATN. This is a form that is considered to be difficult to diagnose due to its rarity and the fact that the symptoms are not usually seen as indicative of trigeminal neuralgia, but more likely causing confusion since they overlap or get mistaken for some other problem. This is one of the reasons why this type is not properly diagnosed or not detected right away. The symptoms associated with ATN are usually mistaken to be a sign of developing migraine headaches, or a symptom that occurs due to a dental problem (such as TMJ or temporo-mandibular joint problems). In other instances, individuals with ATN complaining of its symptoms may get a wrong diagnosis of a musculoskeletal problem or in worse cases, be labeled as a hypochondriac. The labeling of hypochondriasis may occur due to the fact that the pain associated with ATN fluctuates in terms of intensity (individuals with this usually describe pain as either a burning or crushing sensation, mild aching or extremely excruciating), as well as the average time of its presence. In some instances, the pain felt by these individuals with ATN is very much typical to the classic pain felt in the common trigeminal neuralgia problem.

Pre-Trigeminal Type Neuralgia

Deriving from its label, this type of trigeminal neuralgia occurs before the onset of the symptoms of trigeminal neuralgia. However, the symptoms that are experienced by people who have had this were described to be odd or even unrelated to trigeminal neuralgia, or in some cases, seem to be affected by the existence of it. Some reported to have experienced pains in unrelated parts of the face, odd discomforts such as tingling and numbness and even involuntary movement of the affected side of the face.

Multiple Sclerosis Related Type of Trigeminal Neuralgia

Individuals who are affected by this type of neuralgia may present or report symptoms that are usually associated with those being experienced by people diagnosed with typical trigeminal neuralgia. Statistics reveal that there is an approximate 2-4% of all individuals who were diagnosed with trigeminal neuralgia that yielded with positive diagnosis for multiple sclerosis. Moreover, in all individuals who were previously diagnosed with multiple sclerosis, approximately 1% were found to have with trigeminal neuralgia.

People who have been affected with this type of neuralgia are usually younger at the onset of their symptoms as compared to those with the typical neuralgia. Moreover, the pain that they experience has a shorter length of time in progression, but may occur bilaterally.

The main problem in this type of neuralgia lies in the disease process associated with multiple sclerosis itself. Individuals with multiple sclerosis usually manifest with demyelination of the nerves and associated formation of plaques in the brain. Demyelination is a condition where the myelin sheath that acts as a protective covering of the nerves degenerates and is lost. When this happens, the trigeminal nerve and its branches may become affected, leading to the development of neuralgia.

Secondary Type of Neuralgia (Also called Tumor-Related Trigeminal Neuralgia)

The main cause of trigeminal neuralgia is the presence of an injured area in the trigeminal nerve. However, in secondary type of trigeminal neuralgia, the main problem lies with the presence of a lesion or a tumor that causes compression or distortion of the trigeminal nerve. This compression or distortion is responsible for cutting off blood supply to the trigeminal nerve and even injuring the nerve enough to cause pain in the facial muscles. Moreover, individuals affected with this type of neuralgia may also have numbness along the affected facial area, constant aches along the nerve distribution, and even weakness of the associated facial muscles. One of the most common examples of this is the postherpetic or herpetic trigeminal neuralgia, developing after chickenpox or herpes zoster infection.

Although the use of medications proves to be helpful in relieving the symptoms associated with this type of neuralgia, individuals are usually advised to undergo surgeries to address the problem more effectively. The treatment of choice is to remove the tumor surgically to relieve the compression and allow for better blood flow to the trigeminal nerve system. When this happens, there is a very high possibility that the normal functioning of the trigeminal nerve would return and the individual may experience freedom from pain.

Post-Traumatic Trigeminal Neuralgia (Also known as Trigeminal Neuropathy)

This type of trigeminal neuralgia is related to any injury inflicted to the trigeminal nerve that causes severe pain to occur and be experienced by the individual. The most common reasons for this to happen is when the trigeminal nerve gets damaged in a trauma like a motor vehicle accident (the usual cause of trauma in the cranio-facial area), trauma secondary to dental procedures, trauma to the sinuses (usually as complications of surgeries) or even as a complication from a rhizotomy that is performed to treat a previous trigeminal neuralgia of another type.

People who are affected with this condition usually complain of feeling numb in the affected facial region after the suspected injury. This is often followed by pain or sensations around the facial muscles that are similar to phantom pains (the pain felt by amputees on the affected or removed limb) and are called deafferentation pains. This is due to the damage that has occurred to the trigeminal nerve that is beyond repair. Also, this damage is responsible for causing the hyperactive state of the trigeminal nerve nucleus.

Moreover, the pain that is experienced by individuals affected with post-traumatic trigeminal neuralgia is usually constant. It can also be described as being burning or aching in nature and is usually worsened when the individual is exposed to certain triggering factors such as environmental temperatures or air flows. The pain that is related to deafferentation may be experienced by the individual right after the injury to the trigeminal nerve or it may take a few days or even years before it starts. In some instances, individuals who are affected by it may even experience one of the most extreme forms of it called *anesthesia dolorosa*, in which pain that is severe is felt in areas that are found to be totally numb for a prolonged period of time.

The pain that accompanies the diagnosis of post-traumatic trigeminal neuralgia is also quite difficult to manage. In most cases, it has proven to be unresponsive to the use of most pain medications. Other individuals who have had it were also seen to be experiencing more pain in the face when other treatments were carried out that involves stimulation of the affected trigeminal nerve branches.

Failed Trigeminal Neuralgia

This last type of trigeminal neuralgia is applied to individuals who have had histories of having other types of neuralgia who were subjected to the use of various medications to treat the condition, but these drugs prove to be ineffective in managing their pain. This unlucky group of individuals are usually advised to go through a surgical procedure, and then if the pain they are reporting is still persistent after the surgery, they are once again given a round of medications to manage it. The second attempt to use medications intended to manage their pain usually proves to be successful in a majority of individuals and therefore the performance of another surgery is usually no longer necessary. However, there are small numbers of individuals who do not respond positively to almost all forms of management to treat their pain, and are considered to have *failed trigeminal neuralgia.*

A considerable number of those who were diagnosed to have this type may also suffer from additional pain as a result of treatments that are intended to actually cure them of the problem. In some cases, they are found to have traumatic neuralgia as a complication of the numerous surgical interventions done to them such as rhizotomy and microvascular decompression to manage their pain. Due to the nature and unsuccessful response rate of people diagnosed with this type of neuralgia have with the more conservative and widely used treatment methods, the use of other alternative and oftentimes investigational therapies are considered. These therapies include tractotomy or a controlled lesioning in certain parts of the brain stem, pre-motor cortex stimulation (or stimulation of the person's affected brain surface areas), or even the stimulation of the trigeminal nerve itself.

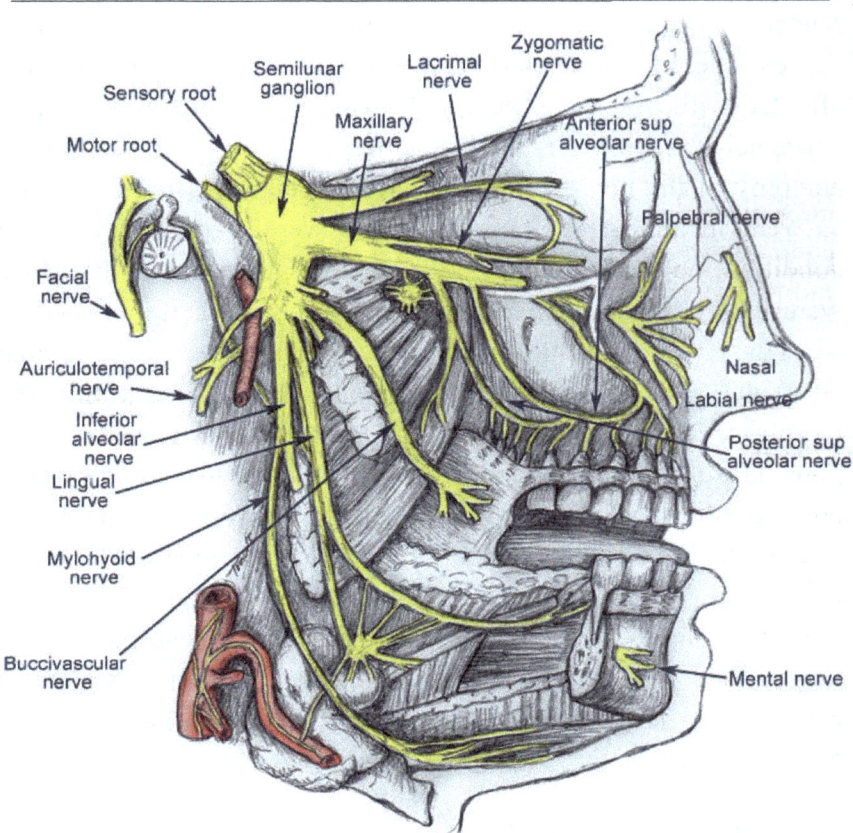

Source: Medscape (Trigeminal Neuralgia)
http://emedicine.medscape.com

4) The Disease Process of Trigeminal Neuralgia

The definitive cause of the presence of trigeminal neuralgia, as mentioned previously in this article, is mostly unknown. This makes it difficult to exactly pinpoint 85% in terms of its pathology. Most pathophysiological presentation of the development of trigeminal neuralgia is based on the etiology related to problems with the central or peripheral trigeminal nerves. The primary reason for the presence of pain in individuals affected with trigeminal neuralgia is the nature of the trigeminal nerve being a sensory nerve. This means that any alteration in the anatomy of the nerve can bring about changes in its functioning as well. In almost 85% of those who were diagnosed with the condition, no lesions along the trigeminal nerve and its branches were found. These were mostly thought to have had the problem secondary to a disruption in the flow of blood to the trigeminal nerve due to compression of the blood vessels. Despite this, the reason for how or why the compression that is mostly seen in the pons is still unknown and therefore related to the idiopathic etiology of trigeminal neuralgia. The compression is often pointed out as the main cause of demyelination (the deterioration of the myelin sheath or the protective covering of the nerves), and the reason for the existence of severe facial pain in most individuals. When these processes occur, the condition is called idiopathic in nature, and is therefore labeled to be the classic form of trigeminal neuralgia.

The presence of any injury into the myelin sheath leads to the exposure of the nerves to its surrounding environment. This exposure increases its risk for subsequent injuries and puts the affected trigeminal nerve and its branches into the pressure of increased stimuli and the interpretation of these stimuli. Most cases of demyelination are seen at the nerves' root entry zone or the REZ, where the transmission of impulses increases and goes beyond the usual capacity of the nerve. Inhibition of impulse transmission is severely compromised due to this condition and sensory stimuli from both inside and the outside environment are greatly amplified even in the face of very subtle stimuli such as mild vibration or even wind breezes brushing into the affected facial areas. This process goes on and on in a vicious cycle, leading to the presence of on-and-off symptoms experienced by individuals diagnosed with trigeminal neuralgia.

"Although a questionable family clustering exists, trigeminal neuralgia (TN) is most likely is multifactorial.

Most cases of trigeminal neuralgia are idiopathic, but compression of the trigeminal roots by tumors or vascular anomalies may cause similar pain, as discussed in Pathophysiology. In one study, 64% of the compressing vessels were identified as an artery, most commonly the superior cerebellar (81%). Venous compression was identified in 36% of cases.

Trigeminal neuralgia is divided into 2 categories, classic and symptomatic. The classic form, considered idiopathic, actually includes the cases that are due to a normal artery present in contact with the nerve, such as the superior cerebellar artery or even a primitive trigeminal artery.

Symptomatic forms can have multiple origins. Aneurysms, tumors, chronic meningeal inflammation, or other lesions may irritate trigeminal nerve roots along the pons causing symptomatic trigeminal neuralgia. An abnormal vascular course of the superior cerebellar artery is often cited as the cause. Uncommonly, an area of demyelination from multiple sclerosis may be the precipitant; lesions in the pons at the root entry zone of the trigeminal fibers have been demonstrated. These lesions may cause a similar pain syndrome as in trigeminal neuralgia."

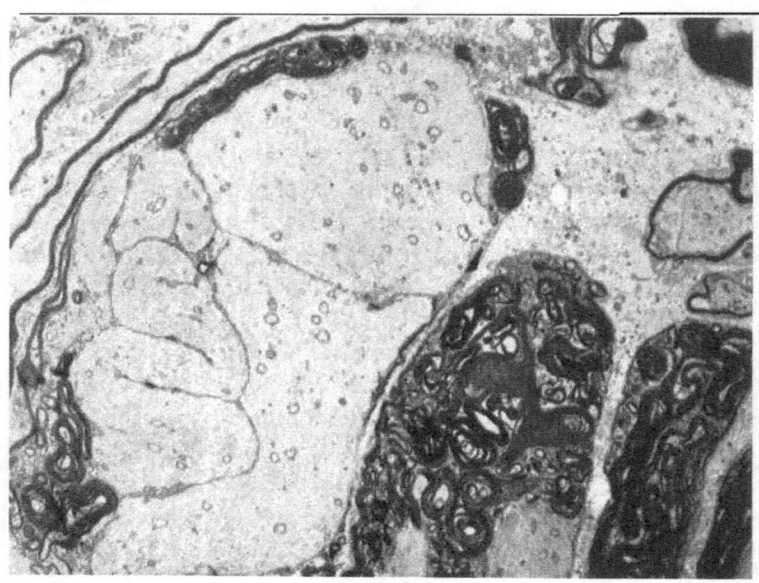

Microscopic demonstration of demyelination in the primary trigeminal neuralgia. Source: Medscape (Trigeminal Neuralgia) http://emedicine.medscape.com

The picture above shows the most plausible reason of the origin (or the etiology) of the chronic disease trigeminal neuralgia.

5) Common Signs and Symptoms of Trigeminal Neuralgia

The main problem with trigeminal neuralgia is the presence of facial pain that varies in terms of its intensity and duration of effect. The typical individual affected with trigeminal neuralgia usually complains of pain that is intense in nature and lasting anywhere from a few seconds to a couple of minutes or even hours, enough to incapacitate them and disrupt their activities of daily living. Aside from the pain usually being intense and with variable duration, it can also occur in a paroxysmal fashion (or come and go), with variable patterns as well. The occurrence of pain is also described by those afflicted with trigeminal neuralgia as having a specific area on their faces that acts as a triggering point (usually referred to as being highly sensitive) that reacts excessively to light touch or air currents. These stimuli act as triggers to start an episode of extreme pain. In some individuals, however, the pain may occur in a spontaneous manner where stimulation to these trigger points are not entirely necessary to cause it. Due to the intensity of the pain and the manner in which it occurs, individuals usually find themselves being unable to carry on their activities of daily living like they used to prior to the diagnosis. They usually find themselves having problems in things such as talking to their friends, eating and enjoying their favorite foods, tooth brushing (either through the use of a manual or electric tooth brush) and even shaving for males. These activities that they were used to do effortlessly before having trigeminal neuralgia usually proves to be painful and difficult to perform. In some individuals, the pain may even be felt along the back of the neck, giving rise to occipital neuralgia and its symptoms.

Moreover, the presence of sounds that are high in pitch, loud noises (such as turning up the radio volume, or being in a concert hall, or in a busy street), chewing and even talking can increase the symptoms felt by some individuals affected by it. They oftentimes complain feeling pain in their faces that are like being stabbed with electric currents, the sensation of their faces being crushed or exploding, or a shooting or burning pain that cannot be relieved by medicines or any other means (intractable).

The pain that is complained by most individuals diagnosed with trigeminal neuralgia attacks only one side of the face more than half of the time. This pain, as previously mentioned, lasts anywhere from a few seconds or minutes, and occurs several times throughout the day. Also, some have even experienced a cyclical occurrence of pain at times, where they have intense pain and alternating cycles of being pain free for a certain period (called remissions) of time before the pain is triggered again in the future. There were findings of some individuals who reported to be on remission or a pain-free period lasting for as long as several month to even years. Also, it has an approximate 10 to 12 percent of individuals with trigeminal neuralgia present with bilateral facial pains. This would them give an indication that the trigeminal nerve systems in both sides of the face have been affected since these nerves are not conjoined and their function is limited only to the side of the face that they are located on. In relation to this, there are also records showing that there are times when trigeminal neuralgia affects one side of the face over a long period of time, there is a possibility that the damage may travel and spread to the other nerve branch as well. In some instances, the inclusion of other nerve branches may go as far as the index finger. Moreover, the attacks of pain experienced by individuals with trigeminal neuralgia can increase in severity or frequency as time goes on.

Systemic involvement of the problem originating from the trigeminal nerve branches may also occur, such as in individuals who were reported to be suffering from multiple sclerosis or in those who have brain tumors that are seen to expand. *Tic convulsive* is one of the most commonly reported problems in this case, where the fifth and seventh cranial nerves are affected simultaneously. In other instances, symptoms may also indicate that the fifth and the ninth cranial nerve areas are the ones that are affected.

Further discussion on the quality of pain as well as the frequency of it was shown in the Trigeminal Neuralgia Clinical Presentation made by Medscape:

"Pain quality

The pain quality is characteristically severe, paroxysmal, and lancinating. It commences with a sensation of electrical shocks in an affected area, then quickly crescendos in less than 20 seconds to an excruciating discomfort felt deep in the face, often contorting the patient's expression. The pain then begins to fade within seconds, only to give way to a burning ache lasting seconds to minutes. During attacks, patients may grimace, wince, or make an aversive head movement, as if trying to escape the pain, thus producing an obvious movement, or tic; hence the term "tic douloureux."

Pain chronicity and frequency

This condition is an exception to the rule that nerve injuries typically produce symptoms of constant pain and allodynia. If the pain is particularly frequent, patients may be difficult to examine during the height of an attack. The number of attacks may vary from less than 1 per day, to a 12 or more per hour, up to hundreds per day. Outbursts fully abate between attacks, even when they are severe and frequent."

Objective assessment of those who are affected with trigeminal nerve problems may also be done by doctors and other members of the health care team. What they usually find out is that in some males who are affected with the problem, they are seen to consciously miss shaving one side of their faces (or the affected side) in an effort to stop the pain or to avoid triggering a pain episode. This is due to the fact that when they experience pain as a result of trigeminal neuralgia, it is usually considered to be debilitating, proving them to be highly incapable of performing activities of daily living independently.

6) Causes of Trigeminal Neuralgia

The main cause of the existence of trigeminal neuralgia that is common among all of its subtypes is the processes of inflammation and associated demyelination of the trigeminal nerve branch. These two, combined with the presence of increased level of sensitivity of the trigeminal nerve is responsible for the condition. The most common causes of these problems may include dental procedures that have gone wrong, infection of the nervous system, diseases that cause demyelination such as multiple sclerosis or conditions that result to compression of the trigeminal nerve that cuts off oxygen and nutrient supply to it. These conditions may also occur in equal number to both male and female patients, most especially in those who are diagnosed to have atypical trigeminal neuralgia.

7) How It Can Affect Me?

Pain is one of the most common symptoms of trigeminal neuralgia. This pain is usually severe in intensity and enough to cause disruptions in a person's capacity to perform activities of daily living. This would render a person sometimes unable to independently carry out his daily activities, leading to an increased sense of having to depend upon others for their needs as well as feelings of inadequacy and unproductiveness. Moreover, as the condition persists, there are also a myriad of other problems that the person manifests with which are not totally related to the root cause of trigeminal nerve injury. In most cases, because of the persistence of severe facial pain, individuals with trigeminal neuralgia also suffer pain during eating, especially as they chew or swallow their food. This causes them to have decreased food intake, leading to nutritional problems and weight loss. Anorexia, or disinterest in eating is also a common problem related to this. In an in-depth study created by Dr. Singh and his colleagues, the prognosis states that:

"After an initial attack, trigeminal neuralgia (TN) may remit for months or even years. Thereafter the attacks may become more frequent, more easily triggered, disabling, and may require long-term medication. Thus, the disease course is typically one of clusters of attacks that wax and wane in frequency. Acute Exacerbations most commonly occur in the fall and spring.

Among the best clinical predictors of a symptomatic form are sensory deficits upon examination and a bilateral distribution of symptoms (but the absence thereof is not a negative predictor). Young age is a moderate predictor, but a fair degree of overlap exists. Lack of therapeutic response and V1 distribution are poor predictors.

Although trigeminal neuralgia is not associated with a shortened life, the morbidity associated with the chronic and recurrent facial pain can be considerable if the condition is not controlled adequately. This condition may evolve into a chronic pain syndrome, and patients may suffer from depression and related loss of daily functioning. Individuals may choose to limit activities that precipitate pain, such as chewing, possibly losing weight in extreme circumstances. In addition, the severity of the pain may lead to suicide.

No laboratory, electrophysiologic, or radiologic testing is routinely indicated for the diagnosis of TN, as patients with a characteristic history and normal neurologic examination may be treated without further workup."

Psychosocial problems are also not uncommon. Due to feelings of inadequacy and inability to become productive in their daily lives, people with trigeminal neuralgia may also suffer from depression. This is because as the pain gets more severe and most treatments prove to be unsuccessful or contribute little help, people get more helpless and powerless to deal with their conditions. Due to this pain also, there are those who have problems speaking because movement of the face as they speak aggravates the pain as well. Furthermore, the isolation that some individuals with the diagnosis put themselves into because of the severity of the pain adds to this problem. Some research has shown that there were cases of people who were diagnosed with the disease that resorted to committing suicide just to end the time that they had to spend dealing with pain. This is the reason why trigeminal neuralgia is also infamously called the "suicide disease".

Facts regarding the frequency in the statistics of the recurrence of the disorder are as follows:

"In 1968, Penman reported the US prevalence of trigeminal neuralgia (TN) as approximately 107 men and 200 women per 1 million people. By 1993, Mauskop noted approximately 40,000 patients have this condition at any particular time, with an incidence of 4-5 cases per 100,000. More recent estimates suggest the prevalence is approximately 1.5 cases per 10,000 populations, with an incidence of approximately 15,000 cases per year.

Rushton and Olafson reported that approximately 1% of patients with multiple sclerosis (MS) develop trigeminal neuralgia, whereas Jensen et al noted that 2% of patients with trigeminal neuralgia have multiple sclerosis, patients with both conditions often have bilateral trigeminal neuralgia.

No geographic tendency or racial differences have been found for trigeminal neuralgia. However, females are affected up to twice as often as males (range, 3:2 to 2:1). In addition, in 90% of patients, the disease begins after 40 years of age, with a typical onset of 60-70 years (middle and later life). Patients who have the disease when aged 20-40 years are more likely to suffer from a demyelinating lesion in the pons secondary to multiple sclerosis; younger patients also tend to have symptomatic or secondary trigeminal neuralgia. There have also been occasional reports of pediatric cases of trigeminal neuralgia.

Another risk factor for this syndrome is hypertension."

Trigeminal Neuralgia as a Symptom

Trigeminal Neuralgia is a disorder but some rare cases show his disease as a symptom to several other more common diseases.

Shingles

The virus that brings chickenpox (*varicella-zoster virus*) causes another underlying infection – shingles (*herpes zoster*). Shingles create a burning pain in the skin along the side of the face and in some case the torso area. After three days, fluid-filled pimples will appear on the skin. The rash that emerged from the tingling area will take another five weeks to recover. Symptoms of shingles include stinging, shooting pain, electric shock and extreme sensitivity to the lightest touch on one side of the face – manifestations also shown in trigeminal neuralgia.

Multiple Sclerosis

The central nervous system throughout the years has had multiple degenerative diseases on the list. Multiple sclerosis (MS) is one of these disabling diseases. Myelin, the sheath that covers nerve fibers in the brain and in the spinal cord are inflamed, destroyed and scarred by the multiple sclerosis. This causes slow reception on the nerve signals, most even block these electrical signals that travel to the eyes and muscles in the body. This disease has varying symptoms that affect almost the whole body. Similar symptoms to the trigeminal neuralgia include tingling facial muscles, slurred speech and difficulty in swallowing.

Brain Tumor

Speech problems are one of the symptoms of having a brain tumor or brain cancer. Trigeminal neuralgia mainly affects the facial nerves and facial functions. Basic human activity such as talking becomes a burden to the person suffering from the disorder.

The symptoms of the trigeminal neuralgia recurs in other known diseases, thus it is safe to say that misdiagnoses of trigeminal neuralgia are unavoidable due to repeating patterns of manifestations on the body.

Ironically, the above mentioned diseases can also cause the trigeminal neuralgia. These diseases, most likely affecting the brain, damage the nerve fibres in the central nervous system and eventually damage the trigeminal nerve.

8) Complications of Trigeminal Neuralgia

Trigeminal Neuralgia is a disease that must never be taken lightly. If not diagnosed early or if misdiagnosed, this could lead to a serious threat in the health of the person. Dr. Singh's study says:

"The chief complication in trigeminal neuralgia is the adverse effects and toxicity experienced routinely with long-term use of anticonvulsant agents. Another complication is the waning efficacy over several years of these drugs in controlling neuralgia, necessitating the addition of a second anticonvulsant, which may cause more drug-related adverse reactions.

Failure to diagnose a brainstem tumor and bone marrow aplasia as an idiosyncratic adverse effect of carbamazepine are common pitfalls to avoid.

Standard care must be applied to invasive procedures, which are most subject to potential claims. Percutaneous neurosurgical procedures and microvascular decompression procedures pose risks of long-term complications. Perioperative risks also exist. Moreover, patients may have to wait for weeks or months after the operation for relief, and some find relief only for 1-2 years and then must weigh the option of a second operation.

Some patients permanently lose sensation over a portion of the face or mouth. Occasionally, patients may suffer jaw weakness and/or corneal anesthesia. Corneal ulceration can result because of trophic disturbances from nerve deafferentation.

After any invasive treatments, reactivation of a herpes simplex infection is not uncommon.

The worst complication is anesthesia dolorosa, an intractable facial dysesthesia, which may be more disabling than the original trigeminal neuralgia. This dysesthesia may be caused by procedures and, sometimes, surgery."

This chronic disorder threatens to disrupt other body functions if not treated early. This can also result to life-changing effects that can alter our routines in life. A chain of failures might occur if not treated properly.

Chapter 2: The History of Trigeminal Neuralgia

Trigeminal neuralgia is not a new disease. This is one condition that has been around for quite a long time. It may have been misdiagnosed in some cases, or was not entirely known at first because of the lack of data. Also, it has been called by another name. This section deals with the existence of trigeminal neuralgia throughout history and some of the most famous personalities who have had to deal with this condition in their lifetimes.

1) Where It All Started?

Trigeminal neuralgia as a condition has been found as early as the first century AD. It was inferred from the manuscripts by Galen and Aretaeus of Cappadocia being described during the early Greek civilizations. It has also been seen written in the notes of Avicenna in the 11th century, called *tortura oris* but it was John Fothergill who was able to accurately describe the condition in 1773. This is the reason for naming the disease after him.

History is teeming with accounts of people who were thought to suffer from trigeminal neuralgia as well. In 1274, an English bishop, Bishop Button, died and was buried in the southern aisle of the cathedral in Wells. He was known to pilgrims and toothache sufferers alike, and was left with offerings at his tomb. The pillars of his tomb were embellished in designed carvings that depict the appearance of people with neuralgia. In 1848, when his sarcophagus was opened by Wilfred Harris, it was found that he has suffered from dental caries, which was considered to be rare during his time. It was then that his condition prior to his death may have been related to trigeminal neuralgia.

In 1671, the German physician Johannes Laurentius Bausch made the most convincing description about trigeminal neuralgia. He is known to have been suffering from a pain in the right side of his face that can be described as lightning-like. This pain rendered him unable to properly eat or speak. He became severely malnourished and emaciated because of this, leading to his death.

Another detailed description about trigeminal neuralgia was made by the famous philosopher and physician John Locke. In his numerous letters to John Mapletoft in 1677, Locke described the condition with reference to a famous patient of his. This patient is the wife of the French ambassador to England, the Countess of Northumberland. However, it was the French physician Nicolas Andre who coined in 1756 the term *tic douloureux* in a book that he entitled *"Observations pratiques sur les maladies de l'urethre et sur plusiers faits convulsifs."* In his book, he has made reference to the presence of facial tics in most patients with the condition, a reason for having the term tic douloureux applied to those diagnosed with the condition, despite the fact that not all patients manifested them.

Together with John Fothergill, Nicolas Andre, Samuel (Fothergill's nephew) and Charles Bell worked on a document that includes an elaborate explanation of the features of patients affected with trigeminal neuralgia, its possible causes, and how to treat it. This document contains Fothergill's description of the condition being *"a painful affection of the face"*, which was later presented in 1773 to the Medical Society of London. He later went on to describe fully the clinical features of the condition we now know as trigeminal neuralgia and one of its most common triggering factors, the introduction of light touch on the affected side of the face. He was also the one who stressed that the condition is more common in women and in those with advancing age. This was confirmed by Pujol in one of his essays. Fothergill himself also suffered from trigeminal neuralgia, as he documented it in a diary in 1804. This diary was entitled *an account of a Painful Affection of the nerves of the Face, commonly called Tic Douloureux.*

2) Famous Personalities Afflicted with the Problem

Trigeminal neuralgia, like all sicknesses and disorders, does not choose who to inflict itself with. The condition, although more commonly seen in the elderly and among women, can affect anyone regardless of their stature in life, age or gender. Cases of trigeminal neuralgia generally occur in the elderly, of 50 years and above. Still, the younger generation is not excluded from the age range. It can happen to anyone of any age, including infancy. Over the years, the condition has gained some spotlight because of the fact that there are famous personalities who were diagnosed with the condition and did not hide the fact that they have trigeminal neuralgia. The following are only some of the most famous personalities who were diagnosed with trigeminal neuralgia.

Melissa Seymour

Melissa Seymour is an Australian author and entrepreneur whose battle with trigeminal neuralgia is public, and therefore well-documented. She was diagnosed to have the condition in 2009 after complaining of severe facial pains for quite some time. After her diagnosis, she underwent a very publicized treatment for the condition in the form of a microvascular decompression surgery.

The entire procedure was covered by various newspapers and magazines from start to finish. She allowed this coverage to happen because she wanted to contribute to raising awareness in the Australian population about trigeminal neuralgia, how it affects people diagnosed with it and the treatment options available to them. Because of this advocacy, the Trigeminal Neuralgia Association of Australia made her one of its patrons.

Truman Capote

Perhaps most notable for his works, the American author Truman Capote is also one of the famous people who have had trigeminal neuralgia. He has battled with the disease in the prime of his career and succumbed to it at the age of 59. The early demise can also be associated with his alcohol problems turned into addiction that he attempted to treat by undergoing rehabilitation.

Salman Khan

One of Bollywood's most famous and talented actors, Salman Khan has made news when he admitted that he has been suffering from trigeminal neuralgia for seven long years prior to making it public. In one of his interviews, he has said that the pain has been severe in the past, prompting him to get treatment but it has not totally gone away. He has complained of pain in his face, along the jaw and gum areas. The disease has also affected his voice box, rendering his voice to become huskier that it originally is. Due to experiencing pain that is unbearable, Khan went to have surgeries abroad to treat his condition.

Chapter 3: What Puts Me At Risk to Develop Trigeminal Neuralgia?

The exact cause as to the existence of trigeminal neuralgia is still largely unknown. This makes it quite a challenge for medical practitioners to effectively prevent it from occurring. Most of the cases of trigeminal neuralgia are associated with a subsequent injury to the trigeminal nerve and its branches. This is what causes the individual suffering from it to report severe pain intensity and other related symptoms. Risk factors for the existence of trigeminal neuralgia may either be classified as modifiable and non-modifiable, depending on their nature. It is worth remembering that these classifications of risk factors are the basis for care planning and prevention of disease occurrence most of the time.

Modifiable risk factors are usually associated with lifestyle and other things that the individual has control over and therefore can change to decrease his risk for the development of the condition. Non-modifiable risk factors, on the other hand, are those that the individual has no control over and therefore cannot be changed. This category of risk factor only helps in the planning of the prevention of the disease by ensuring those conditions and other things that can potentiate its capacity to cause the occurrence of a disease is minimized.

1) Modifiable Risk Factors

Most of the modifiable risk factors that bring about the occurrence of trigeminal neuralgia in most people are related to an injury inflicted upon the trigeminal nerve and its branches.

One of the most commonly associated factors to the existence of the problem is damage to the trigeminal nerve that is secondary to an ineffective blood and oxygen supply to the trigeminal nerve. Cigarette smoking can bring about this condition, especially if the individual has been smoking for a prolonged period of time. The nicotine in the cigarette smoke when inhaled causes a reaction of the endocrine glands, increasing the production and release of epinephrine. This increased level of epinephrine causes the constriction of blood vessels, decreasing the efficiency of blood flow to numerous parts of the body including the trigeminal nerve.

Infection with the herpes virus may also lead to the development of trigeminal neuralgia. This can cause inflammation of the trigeminal nerve and may last until the person is treated effectively. When a person develops trigeminal neuralgia because of this risk factor, treatment using the same types of drugs used for herpes-related infections may be chosen.

Other modifiable triggers or risk factors associated with the attack of trigeminal neuralgia may include the presence of bright car lights, loud sounds, high levels of tensions or stress, and even poor dietary choices. Among this group of triggers, it is worth to note that improvement of a person's dietary intake or status may prove to be both a preventive and treatment as well, since a person with trigeminal neuralgia may also exhibit poor nutritional intake because of severe facial pain and nausea associated with the disease.

2) Non-Modifiable Risk Factors

One of the most notable non-modifiable risk factors associated with the presence of trigeminal neuralgia is age. It has been noted that most of trigeminal neuralgia cases appear and are diagnosed when a person reaches the age of 50 and above. In addition to this, degenerative changes to the nerves occur in the advanced aged population so putting them to increased risk to develop injury to the trigeminal nerve. Since increased numbers of cases of trigeminal neuralgia are also diagnosed among women, gender can also be said as a risk factor.

3) Is trigeminal neuralgia hereditary?

This is one of the most common questions that are asked in associated with the condition and the answer to it is still not entirely clear. Experts say that most of the cases of trigeminal neuralgia are not hereditary although 17% of cases of bilateral trigeminal neuralgia and 4.1% of unilateral trigeminal neuralgia have trigeminal neuralgia in their close relatives.

4) Association between Trigeminal Neuralgia and Cluster Headaches

The life of a person diagnosed with trigeminal neuralgia is drastically changed because of the presence of the condition. On top of the severe facial pains and the presence of difficulty in interpreting sensations on the affected parts of the face where the trigeminal nerve traverses, the individual might also feel another group of syndromes referred to as cluster headaches. These headaches are described mostly to occur on one side of the face, and usually originate behind the eye. The pain felt by the individual is excruciating in nature and gets affected by the person's sleeping patterns. The presence of cluster headaches is triggered by an attack of trigeminal neuralgia, and likewise, the attack of trigeminal neuralgia in some people is affected by the presence of cluster headache symptoms.

Chapter 4: How is Trigeminal Neuralgia Diagnosed?

Until now, there are no definitive laboratory tests or work-up that can fully and specifically assess the presence of trigeminal neuralgia in an individual. Other testing procedures, such as radiologic or electrophysiologic in nature, are not usually prescribed for individuals suffering from trigeminal neuralgia to undergo. In most cases, the current health history, development of symptoms and a routine neurologic assessment is enough to lead a physician to pronounce the diagnosis of trigeminal neuralgia. The diagnosis is mainly based on the presence of severe facial pain that is complained by almost all individuals suffering from it. This minimizes or eliminates entirely the necessity of a laboratory test is some instances.

1) Invasive Diagnostic Testing Procedures

However, there is still routine testing that is carried out not to diagnose the presence of trigeminal neuralgia per se, but other conditions that may be the underlying cause or even complication of trigeminal neuralgia. Tests such as blood counts or liver function studies may be done, especially if the use of anti-convulsant agents such as carbamazepine is being considered by the physician. Regular monitoring of blood sodium levels may also be necessary to carry out when other types of anti-convulsant drugs such as oxcarbazepine are prescribed since it can cause severe reduction of this in some individuals.

Diagnostic tests done in most individuals suffering from trigeminal neuralgia may either be non-invasive or invasive, depending on their nature. These tests do not specifically pinpoint the presence of trigeminal neuralgia, but may help in identifying the root cause of the condition. Tests for diseases such as systemic lupus erythematosus and scleroderma may be done, since their conditions have often been linked to the presence of trigeminal neuralgia in individuals with atypical presentation of the condition. Blood work drawn up in this testing usually includes the erythrocyte sedimentation rate or ESR, complete blood counts or CBC and those that are definitive or indicative of the presence of SLE or scleroderma like the antinuclear antibody (ANA) and other antibody tests.

Analysis of the CSF or cerebrospinal fluid may also be performed when a possible cancer metastasis is pointed out to be the cause of the problem with the trigeminal nerve. The test may also determine the type of preparation needed in case the individual needs to undergo surgeries to treat the condition. Moreover, in some individuals who are beyond 60 years of age, some doctors opt to diagnose the presence of trigeminal neuralgia in a different manner. These individuals are those who are usually given the diagnosis of trigeminal neuralgia of idiopathic nature. What is being done to these individuals is that they are given a dosage of an anti-convulsant drug such as carbamazepine and their response to its administration is assessed. Those who receive the idiopathic trigeminal neuralgia diagnosis are those who usually report or experience relief of symptoms after the drug is administered.

In some individuals whose facial muscles are also affected by the presence of trigeminal nerve injury, an electromyelogram may be performed. This test involves the insertion of needles into the affected muscles of the face and evaluating the electrical activity of these muscles. The EMG is usually performed to see if the lack of facial muscle movement is due to a neurologic cause or just the apprehension of the individual to move his facial muscles because of the fear of triggering pain. The discomfort that comes along with the procedure is remedied by administration of local anesthetics to the area prior to the testing.

2) Non-Invasive Diagnostic Procedures

The usual non-invasive diagnostic procedures taken for individuals who are diagnosed with trigeminal neuralgia consist of imaging studies. These are performed to assess the trigeminal nerve and to ascertain the location of the damage or injury and how far it extends to other structures inside the brain. Lesions and tumors are usually seen on these studies, and their exact size can also be determined.

Magnetic resonance imaging studies, or MRI, is one of the most common imaging studies performed to determine the diagnosis of trigeminal neuralgia. This test is performed to determine if there is a presence of compression (usually caused by tumors) along the trigeminal nerve and its branches. The process by which MRI creates an image of the trigeminal nerve is defined by the use of radio waves and strong magnetic field activities. This allows the MRI to search beyond the cranium and into the brain, extending to the trigeminal nerve itself. Apart from being non-invasive, the MRI also helps in ruling out other possible conditions leading to the development of facial pain that may or may not be related to the diagnosis of trigeminal neuralgia.

Another study that is also undertaken is CT scanning. Like the MRI, this is also an imaging study that can provide visualization of the affected trigeminal nerve and its branches. This imaging study takes pictures of several areas of the brain and even some parts of the face where the trigeminal nerve travels. Unlike the MRI, the CT scan provides monochromatic images, but is relatively helpful in arriving at a correct diagnosis of the condition. Most of the CT scan results are presented in a plate of 6 or more images of the trigeminal nerve and its area of distribution.

3) Tests for Trigeminal Neuralgia

Other than performing tests using either invasive or non-invasive diagnostic tools, there are also assessment parameters that can be used for the person suffering from attacks of severe and debilitating pain caused by trigeminal neuralgia. These tests can be done at the physicians' clinic and are used as baseline assessment information in diagnosing the presence of trigeminal neuralgia. However, the findings of these tests alone are not sufficient to support a diagnosis of trigeminal neuralgia and would still have to be corroborated with the results of the diagnostic tests mentioned in the previous sections.

Examinations for both the motor and sensory functioning of the trigeminal nerve are essential to carry out to check the degree of involvement and limitation in the functioning of the nerve occurs when trigeminal neuralgia is suspected. Usually, prior to the performance of the test, the individual is asked to assume a comfortable position and to relax. This ensures that there is no additional muscle tension that can result in a false-positive finding. Since most of these tests require that the individual follow commands from the physician or nurse performing the test, it is important that his or her full cooperation is gained before the test starts. Explaining the test and how important it is to help in diagnosis usually resolves this issue.

In assessing the motor functioning of the individual, the examiner normally observes for the presence of normal facial muscle activity. This means that most of its actions are controlled by the individual at will, or what is termed as involuntary. Expected normal findings would include no occurrence of facial muscle tremors, no involuntary movements resembling chewing motion or no presence of trismus or spasms (tonic contractions in other literatures) of the jaw muscles. Movement of the jaw is also assessed for, as well as the ability of the individual to open and close it as he or she clenches the teeth. Moreover, the movements should also be symmetrical, meaning that they appear equally on either sides of the face. Abnormal motor functioning of the trigeminal nerve would return with results indicating paralysis, other than the pain that is usually associated with trigeminal neuralgia. Findings would include deviation of the jaw to the affected side of the face when the mouth is opened, and presence of misaligned teeth in the front (central medial incisors) when the individual is asked to clench his jaw.

Sensory functioning of the trigeminal nerve is also assessed. This would include the examiner checking the sensitivity of the trigeminal nerve branches in the areas of the face such as the cheeks, the oral mucosa (the area inside the mouth), jaw and even the forehead. These areas should not have any pain or problems in terms of their ability to distinguish and interpret sensations. Any findings outside the expected norms are reported and are being used as a reference to see if the individual is to be diagnosed with trigeminal neuralgia.

Reflexes are also assessed along the face to determine the combined sensory and motor function of the trigeminal nerve in the jaw and cornea. The test used when examining the jaw is the Jaw Jerk reflex (also referred to as mandibular reflex in other

45

literature). Corneal reflex is also assessed. In this, the examiner uses a cotton wisp to lightly touch the cornea of the eyes of the person being examined. A normal finding would be elicited when the individual exhibits blinking of both eyes, indicating that there is the presence of a consensual reflex.

The Clinical Study of Trigeminal Neuralgia gave a list of the very blatant signs and symptoms of a person who has this chronic disease:

Signs and symptoms

TN presents as attacks of stabbing unilateral facial pain, most often on the right side of the face. The number of attacks may vary from less than 1 per day to 12 or more per hour and up to hundreds per day.

Triggers of pain attacks include the following:

- *Chewing, talking, or smiling*
- *Drinking cold or hot fluids*
- *Touching, shaving, brushing teeth, blowing the nose*
- *Encountering cold air from an open automobile window*

Pain localization is as follows:

- *Patients can localize their pain precisely*
- *The pain commonly runs along the line dividing either the mandibular and maxillary nerves or the mandibular and ophthalmic portions of the nerve*
- *In 60% of cases, the pain shoots from the corner of the mouth to the angle of the jaw*
- *In 30%, pain jolts from the upper lip or canine teeth to the eye and eyebrow, sparing the orbit itself*

- *In less than 5% of cases, pain involves the ophthalmic branch of the facial nerve*

The pain has the following qualities:

- *Characteristically severe, paroxysmal, and lancinating*
- *Commences with a sensation of electrical shocks in the affected area*
- *Crescendos in less than 20 seconds to an excruciating discomfort felt deep in the face, often contorting the patient's expression*
- *Begins to fade within seconds, only to give way to a burning ache lasting seconds to minutes*
- *Pain fully abates between attacks, even when they are severe and frequent*
- *Attacks may provoke patients to grimace, wince, or make an aversive head movement, as if trying to escape the pain, thus producing an obvious movement, or tic; hence the term "tic douloureux"*

Other diagnostic clues are as follows:

- *Patients carefully avoid rubbing the face or shaving a trigger area, in contrast to other facial pain syndromes, in which they massage the face or apply heat or ice*
- *Many patients try to hold their face still while talking, to avoid precipitating an attack*
- *In contrast to migrainous pain, attacks of TN rarely occur during sleep"*

The signs and symptoms of the disease also have different levels. It is important to know the levels of pain the patient is suffering.

There are certain parameters Dr. Singh's team has set which is elaborated below:

"Strict criteria for TN as defined by the International Headache Society (IHS) are as follows:

- *A – Paroxysmal attacks of pain lasting from a fraction of a second to 2 minutes, affecting 1 or more divisions of the trigeminal nerve and fulfilling criteria B and C*
- *B – Pain has at least 1 of the following characteristics: (1) intense, sharp, superficial or stabbing; or (2) precipitated from trigger areas or by trigger factors*
- *C – Attacks stereotyped in the individual patient*
- *D – No clinically evident neurologic deficit*
- *E – Not attributed to another disorder*

IHS criteria for symptomatic TN vary slightly from the strict criteria and include the following:

- *A – Paroxysmal attacks of pain lasting from a fraction of a second to 2 minutes, with or without persistence of aching between paroxysms, affecting 1 or more divisions of the trigeminal nerve and fulfilling criteria B and C*
- *B – Pain has at least 1 of the following characteristics: (1) intense, sharp, superficial or stabbing; or (2) precipitated from trigger areas or by trigger factors*
- *C – Attacks stereotyped in the individual patient*
- *D – A causative lesion, other than vascular compression, demonstrated by special investigations and/or posterior fossa exploration*

A blood count and liver function tests are required if therapy with carbamazepine is contemplated. Oxcarbazepine can cause hyponatremia, so the serum sodium level should be measured after institution of therapy."

Chapter 5: Treating Trigeminal Neuralgia

The presence of trigeminal nerve injury and the symptoms it brings along with it makes it necessary for it to be treated as soon as it is diagnosed. This also ensures that the symptoms will not worsen, and at the same time, develop into complications such as depression and other psychosocial and physical problems. Treatment options may range from the more conservative use of medications to the more aggressive surgical interventions if medications did not bring about satisfactory management of the condition.

In MedScape's in-depth review on trigeminal neuralgia, they presented in bullet forms some treatment they have deemed effective in the treatment of the disorder.

"Trigeminal neuralgia is treated on an outpatient basis, unless neurosurgical intervention is required. Management of this condition must be tailored individually, based on the patient's age and general condition. In the case of symptomatic trigeminal neuralgia, adequate treatment is that of its cause, the details of which are out of the scope of this article.

Because most patients incur trigeminal neuralgia when older than 60 years, medical management is the logical initial therapy. Medical therapy is often sufficient and effective, allowing surgical consideration only if pharmacologic treatment fails. Medical therapy alone is adequate treatment for 75% of patients.

Patients may find immediate and satisfying relief with one medication, typically carbamazepine. However, because this disorder may remit spontaneously after 6-12 months, patients may elect to discontinue their medication in the first year following the diagnosis. Most must restart medication in the future. Furthermore, over the years, they may require a second or third drug to control breakthrough episodes and finally may need surgical intervention.

Simpler, less invasive procedures are well tolerated but usually provide only short-term relief. At this point, further and perhaps more invasive operations may be required, and with these procedures the risk of the disabling adverse effect of anesthesia dolorosa increases.

Thus, treatment can be subdivided into pharmacologic therapy, percutaneous procedures, surgery, and radiation therapy. Adequate pharmacologic trials should always precede the contemplation of a more invasive approach.

Transcranial magnetic stimulation appears promising, but results are still scarce.

Treatment of TN comprises the following:

- *Pharmacologic therapy*
- *Percutaneous procedures (eg, percutaneous retrogasserian glycerol rhizotomy)*
- *Surgery (eg, microvascular decompression)*
- *Radiation therapy (i.e., gamma knife surgery)*

Features of pharmacologic therapy are as follows:

- *Pharmacologic trials should always precede the contemplation of a more invasive approach, as medical therapy alone is adequate treatment for 75% of patients*

- *Single-drug therapy may provide immediate and satisfying relief*
- *Carbamazepine is the best studied drug for TN and the only one with US Food and Drug Administration (FDA) approval for this indication*
- *Because TN may remit spontaneously after 6-12 months, patients may elect to discontinue their medication in the first year following the diagnosis; most must restart medication in the future*
- *Over the years, patients may require a second or third drug to control breakthrough episodes and finally may need surgical intervention*
- *Lamotrigine and baclofen are second-line therapies*
- *Controlled data for adding a second drug when the first fails exist only for the addition of lamotrigine to carbamazepine*
- *Gabapentin has demonstrated effectiveness in TN, especially in patients with multiple sclerosis.*

Features of surgical treatment include the following:

- *Three operative strategies now prevail: percutaneous procedures, gamma knife surgery (GSK), and microvascular decompression (MVD)*
- *Ninety percent of patients are pain-free immediately or soon after any of the operations, but the relief is much more long-lasting with microvascular decompression*
- *Percutaneous surgeries make sense for older patients with medically unresponsive trigeminal neuralgia*
- *Younger patients and those expected to do well under general anesthesia should first consider microvascular decompression."*

1) Medical Management

The use of medications for trigeminal neuralgia is implemented not only in terms of managing its root cause and the symptoms, but also in the prevention of complications as well. Pain relief is the main thrust for the use of medications, since this symptom is the major complaint of almost all individuals diagnosed with trigeminal neuralgia.

Anti-Convulsant Drugs

Medications such as carbamazepine, a known anti-convulsant, have been used as the first-line treatment option for people diagnosed with trigeminal neuralgia. This is due to the nature of facial pain seen in people with trigeminal neuralgia that resembles seizure activities. However, some practitioners avoid using carbamazepine because it is associated with a number of side effects and other adverse reactions. This is remedied by the use of other anti-convulsant medications like gabapentin.

The use of these medications alone may prove to be effective to some patients, relieving pain and minimizing the need for other therapies. However, it should be important to assess the individual's complete health history and the presenting signs and symptoms of the disease be fully assessed so that effective therapy may be given.

Tricyclic Anti-Depressant

There are instances when the uses of anti-seizure drugs are not effective for treating the pain associated with trigeminal neuralgia. Medications of other classification or category may also be used. Tricyclic anti-depressants may then be used for this purpose. These medications may include common drugs of this category such as nortriptyline and amitriptyline.

The use of anti-depressants in the treatment of individuals with trigeminal neuralgia is considered dual action. The primary intention of its use in trigeminal neuralgia is for the achievement of relief of neuropathic pain, while it's ideally intended use is for managing depression. Also, anti-depressants can be used as part of multiple drug therapy in some individuals who are given other types of medications as well.

Opioid Drugs

In some instances when the use of other less potent drugs prove to be ineffective in managing the pain, opioids may be prescribed to ensure that pain is managed and the individual is able to carry on individual performance of his activities of daily living. Drugs such as oxycodone or morphine may be given in addition to other drugs like anti-convulsants to achieve optimum pain relief. Due to the high potency of these drugs, most individuals who are given treatment regimens having opioids as part of it have their pain and other related symptoms managed so well that they barely require the use of other more aggressive treatment options. However, the use of these medications may require caution, since opioids are known to cause psychological dependence or addiction.

Use of Other Drugs

In individuals who are diagnosed specifically to be affected with trigeminal neuralgia as a complication of herpes-virus infection, topical medications may be prescribed for them to use. Preparations in the form of ointments or creams are to be applied to the affected trigeminal nerve branch such as gallium maltolate.

2) Surgical Interventions

In some instances when the use of medications to treat trigeminal neuralgia prove to be not as effective in pain management and relief of other associated problems, doctors would prescribe the individual to undergo surgical procedures to treat the condition.

According to the information from the Patient (UK), surgery for trigeminal neuralgia falls under two categories:

"Decompression surgery

This means an operation to relieve the pressure on the trigeminal nerve. As mentioned earlier, most cases of TN are due to a blood vessel in the brain pressing on the trigeminal nerve as it leaves the skull. An operation can ease the pressure from the blood vessel (decompress the nerve) and therefore ease symptoms. This operation has the best chance of long-term relief of symptoms. However, it is a major operation involving a general anesthetic and brain surgery to get to the root of the nerve within the brain. Although usually successful, there is a small risk of serious complications, such as a stroke or deafness, following this operation. A very small number of people have died as a result of this operation.

Ablative surgical treatments

Ablative means to destroy. There are various procedures that can be used to destroy the root of the trigeminal nerve and thus ease symptoms. For example, one procedure is called stereotactic radio-surgery (gamma knife surgery). This uses radiation targeted at the trigeminal nerve root to destroy the nerve root. The advantage of these ablative procedures is that they can be done much more easily than decompression surgery, as they do rot involve formal brain surgery. So, there is much less risk of serious complications or death than there is with decompression surgery. However, there is more of a risk that you will be left with a lack of sensation in a part of your face or eye, as the treatment may mean that the trigeminal nerve will not function normally again. Also, there is a higher chance that the symptoms will return at some stage in the future, compared with decompression surgery. The chance of a cure from both decompression and ablative treatments is good. But, there are pros and cons of each. If you are considering surgery, the advice from a specialist is essential to help you decide which procedure is best for you."

On a much deeper level, there are specific surgeries that a patient can choose from. Over the years of research, doctors and specialists from the medical field have created a number of offers to relieve the pains of people suffering from trigeminal neuralgia.

Microvascular Decompression

One of the reasons for the existence of trigeminal nerve injury, and consequently, trigeminal neuralgia, is blockage in the microcirculation leading to the nerve itself. Due to this, one of the most effective therapies that can also bring about lasting effects when performed is the microvascular decompression procedure. In this treatment option, the compression that extends itself into the trigeminal nerve, such as a tumor or other causes of injury, is being separated and lifted off the trigeminal nerve. After this, blood flow to the trigeminal nerve and its branches is improved by padding those that are near to the affected nerves. These are usually located below the cranium in the brainstem itself.

Rhizotomy

If the individual would not be a good candidate for the performance of microvascular decompression, another procedure might be performed to relieve pain associated with trigeminal neuralgia. Rhizotomy is one of those procedures usually performed on individuals suffering from trigeminal neuralgia. This procedure, although performed on a different set of processes, promises similar results to that of microvascular decompression. The main principle being employed in this procedure is the induction of a lesion along the specific nerve branches and their distribution lines along the trigeminal nerve and travels down to the brainstem. These lesions are created or put in place to allow interruption pf pain impulse transmission and to render a moderate responsiveness of the nerves, making them less sensitive.

There are several forms of rhizotomy. Radiofrequency guided rhizotomy is most frequently performed, since this has a bigger success rate. Other forms such as the Cyber Knife (also known as the Gamma Knife) are also used, wherein radiation is used to perform the surgery, eliminating the need for an actual surgical incision. There is also glycerol rhizotomy and balloon compression rhizotomy. However, these forms are not often used to treat trigeminal neuralgia since they have lower rates of effectiveness. Another form, percutaneous radiofrequency thermorhizotomy, is also used since it has the same effectiveness as the use of the Gamma Knife, but this may require several treatments to be done, as its effectiveness on the operated trigeminal nerve may decrease as time passes.

The most commonly used rhizotomy procedures are listed below:

1. *Percutaneous Glycerol Rhizotomy.*

In this rhizotomy technique, glycerol, a chemical liquid which is clear, is injected into the area affected with trigeminal neuralgia. The procedure is usually performed by introducing a local anesthetic into the operative site, rendering the individual aware of the entire procedure without feeling any pain. In some cases, however, the use of general anesthesia or IV sedation may be employed when the individual prefers it over local anesthesia. Then a needle measuring approximately 3.5 inches (G 20 spinal needle in most cases) is introduced in the affected area besides the face (this usually is the skin on the side of the mouth) and is guided to reach the opening found on the base of the skull. This step involves the needle passing through the foramen ovale (the opening found in the base of the skull leading to the spinal cord). After this, a dye is introduced into the area while images are taken via an x-ray machine to confirm proper placement of the needle. Since most dyes and contrast media use iodine as its base, the presence of allergies with iodine needs to be ruled out first. After checking proper placement, the glycerol can now be introduced into the space that is around the Gasserion ganglion. The introduction of the glycerol stimulates a process that injures the trigeminal nerve minimally, decreasing the severity of pain, while having decreased risk to render permanent numbness to the facial muscles. The procedure is not entirely successful, despite relative pain relief after the treatment. This is because most of those who underwent glycerol rhizotomy usually have pain recurrence a few years after the treatment, necessitating for a repeat procedure or the performance of other therapies to reduce pain.

2. Percutaneous Balloon Compression Rhizotomy.

This procedure is an alternative technique when the performance of a percutaneous trigeminal rhizotomy alone is not sufficient to relieve pain in those who opted for it. In this therapy, a balloon compression operation is performed to potentiate the pain-relieving effects of a percutaneous trigeminal rhizotomy. In the performance of this surgery, the individual is usually placed under the effect of general anesthesia, and then a needle is introduced under the facial skin and is advanced and guided to reach the Gasserion ganglion. This needle is larger bore so that a balloon can be fitted inside it and be inflated later on. Once the needle reaches its desired position, the balloon is then inflated, causing injury to the root of the trigeminal nerve and the Gasserion ganglion to render pain reduction. Most of those undergoing this procedure complain of pain located in the upper part of the face. When this surgery is performed, the risk of rendering loss of sensation to the cornea is minimized when injuring the trigeminal nerve. People who undergo this procedure however should know that there are temporary side effects associated with injuring the trigeminal nerve, such as the weakening of the facial muscles responsible for chewing. Moreover, the numbness along the face felt by individuals after this procedure is more than what is felt when a glycerol rhizotomy is done.

3. Radiofrequency Rhizotomy.

This is another percutaneous rhizotomy procedure when other procedures are not successful or cannot be performed to those suffering from trigeminal neuralgia. In this therapy, individuals are kept awake throughout the procedure. This is because ongoing assessment about the numbing effect of the radiofrequency-produced lesion needs to be performed on the individual. The procedure is performed through the use of a specialized electrode emitting radiofrequency that is surgically introduced into the trigeminal pathway into the face and is led to the Gasserion ganglion. After the position is confirmed, mild electrical impulses are run through the electrodes, which cause tingling sensations along the face of the individual. After this, the electrode's temperature is increased, heating it so that the nerve can be injured. These are all done while the individual receives strong sedatives. One of the advantages of this form of rhizotomy is that it can provide long-term pain relief. This has been found to occur in almost two-thirds of all individuals who received it, with pain relief averaging to five years or more. Despite this positive information about this procedure, there is still a need to research more on the relative long-term side effects such as permanent numbness of the face. Also, in some individuals, reports of anesthesia dolorosa may occur. This condition is characterized by facial numbness with co-existing severe pains.

4. Microsurgical Rhizotomy.

This is a relatively phased-out rhizotomy procedure that involves the opening up of the location of the affected trigeminal nerve branch through a surgical incision and removing it to provide pain relief. This was done more than a few decades ago, most especially when the trigeminal nerve branch located in the lower side of the face, or V_3, is responsible for the painful sensations. However, microsurgical rhizotomy was replaced by other non-aggressive procedures such as percutaneous rhizotomy and microvascular decompression procedures. This surgery is still performed on rare instances like the preference of the individual for it or when less invasive procedures are deemed to be ineffective. One advantage that this surgery has over the other therapies is that numbness of the lower portions of the face is usually localized to the area being operated on.

5. *Gamma Knife Radio-surgery.*

The use of this technique is one of the most complicated of all rhizotomy procedures, since it employs the use of focused beam radiation via an MRI machine together with the surgery. This is considered as a form of laser treatment for those who are diagnosed with trigeminal neuralgia. However, the means for pain relief employed in this surgery is the same for the other forms, and that is injuring the affected trigeminal nerve branch to render pain relief to the individual. This starts with the application of a frame around the person's head and taking MRI images before an instrument known as the Gamma Knife is introduced. This instrument directs an approximate 201 focused cobalt radiation beams into the root of the trigeminal nerve. This step causes the trigeminal nerve to suffer injuries over an extended period of time, varying from a few days to a few weeks, causing a delay in the pain relief reports. Because of this, the procedure can render longer pain-free episodes. The use of the radiation should be controlled when Gamma Knife Radio-surgery is performed because higher doses can increase the risk of facial numbness and even paralysis. Since this treatment is relatively new, most doctors are still adamant in performing it due to the limited research studies conducted on its efficiency over time and the costs that doing it would incur to those suffering from trigeminal neuralgia.

Neurectomy

This procedure in the treatment of trigeminal neuralgia was first attempted during the 18th century when affected trigeminal nerve branches were operated on, with limited success into the procedure. This treatment method is now usually done in the clinics and in hospitals by a surgeon known as a maxillofacial surgeon. Neurectomy is not widely reported, and their advantages in the treatment of individuals with rendering pain relief is therefore not known to most people. This therapy has been the topic of some research studies, with its ability to render pain relief in over 80% of individuals who were diagnosed with typical trigeminal neuralgia symptoms.

Neurectomy can be performed more than once in some individuals who experience recurrent pains, with subsequent treatments having a high success rate. This makes it a good treatment option for those who have tried other therapies with limited success rates. However, since there is limited source of information as to the advantages and disadvantages of this treatment option, the possibility of suffering from any adverse reaction after therapy and risk of not having successful treatment should also be considered.

The process in which neurectomy is done starts with a surgical cut or incision done at the area of the supra-orbital nerve located in the eyebrow, or in the infra-orbital, lingual and alveolar nerves that can be located inside the mouth of the individual. An avulsion or a tearing away of the affected nerve branch is done through the help of endoscopic equipment, where the affected nerves are divided as well. Any openings are blocked using plugs or surgical wax preparations and the remaining portions of the trigeminal nerve may be cauterized to enhance the effectiveness of the treatment.

Cryotherapy

Another surgical procedure that can be used in the treatment of trigeminal neuralgia is cryotherapy. This is a procedure that uses a device called a cryoprobe. This device has a tip that can go to temperatures as low as -50 to -70 centigrade, and is applied to a peripheral branch of the affected trigeminal nerve to freeze it.

This freezing of the nerve is what renders pain relief in those who have used it to treat trigeminal neuralgia.

In this procedure, the individual is normally placed under general anesthesia or IV sedation. Then the cryoprobe is introduced to the affected trigeminal nerve branch and freezing starts. This procedure, because of its simplicity and limited tissue damage associated with it, is tolerated well by most individuals. However, there is a need to repeat the procedure for some because of the limited time (usually ranges from 6, 12 or 18 months) that the procedure renders painless episodes to those who underwent through it. There are also individuals who underwent the procedure who experienced pain in another branch of the trigeminal nerve, or need to continue intake of medications to manage pain. Moreover, when cryosurgery is performed, there is the risk of developing infection in the operated areas, but this can be managed through the use of antibiotics. Due to the presence of more disadvantages over the apparent temporary advantages of this treatment many physicians do not recommend cryosurgery for trigeminal neuralgia treatment. One of the primary reasons for the use of this therapy is when other surgical interventions or the use of radiation-based treatments cannot be performed on the person suffering from trigeminal neuralgia.

Peripheral Trigeminal Nerve Blocks, Sectioning and Avulsions

These groups of surgeries are usually reserved for those individuals with trigeminal neuralgia who have high risks of developing complications when other procedures are done. These groups of individuals include those who are very old, weak, or those who have medical conditions that contraindicate the performance of other therapies to treat trigeminal neuralgia. Peripheral nerve blocks, sectioning and avulsions of the trigeminal nerve are performed to directly cause injury to the trigeminal nerve and its branches that exit from the skull, in the linings of the mouth, or beneath the skin of the face. The injury is caused through the introduction of an oxidizing substance (usually alcohol), cutting off or tearing away (avulsion) of the affected trigeminal nerve branches. The procedure has a relatively quick pain-relief time frame, despite the temporary numbness experienced by the individual in the affected areas. However, there are instances in which the numbness becomes severe or affects the entire face. Because of the possibility of pain recurrence, interventions involving these procedures are usually done repeatedly if long-term pain relief is targeted. Moreover, other more permanent pain-relief procedures may also be considered.

Alcohol Blocks

The use of the alcohol block procedure for the management of pain associated with trigeminal nerve damage has been around since the last century. Basically, alcohol blocks are used and applied on the peripheral and ganglionic portions of the trigeminal nerve to render pain relief. One thing about alcohol blocks is that the technique in its performance is highly similar to procedures involving the ablation of the peripheral nerves. Despite its long time being used and practiced, there are some physicians questioning its use and advantage because of the occurrence of adverse effects. Because the treatment is easy to perform, there are still those that advocate its use for therapy in individuals with trigeminal neuralgia.

Theoretically speaking, alcohol block procedure is easy to perform. The treatment employs the direct administration of injections consisting of alcohol solutions into the affected trigeminal nerve and its branches directly. This step is usually associated with pain and development of swelling (or edema) in the tissues surrounding the area being treated. However, the presence of swelling in the area surrounding the nerve being treated can lead to unaesthetic results, excluding alcohol block procedure from being one of treatments of choice. Most individuals undergoing this procedure are those who are frail, not fit for other more aggressive medical procedures, or those who specifically chose this procedure as a treatment for their trigeminal neuralgia.

Other Procedures

Apart from the two most widely used procedures mentioned above, there are still three more therapies that are invasive in nature used in the treatment of trigeminal neuralgia. These therapies include the use of catheters and needles, which are surgically inserted into the affected facial area where the trigeminal nerve splits into its three branches. These are guided by a fiber-optic tube that allows the physician performing it to see the area operated on from a monitor. Balloon compression procedure is one of the therapies that is performed percutaneously with high success rates, especially among elderly patients who experience recurrence of pain after a microvascular decompression procedure.

Corrosion of the nerve fibers is used when other therapies were not successful in achieving pain relief. This can be done through injecting a glycerol solution. The solution is introduced in an area near the junction of the nerves responsible for pain, which inflicts injury on these nerves that allows it control pain impulse signals.

Studies are being conducted to see which surgery is best for the chronic disorder. In an article in Medscape, they put to account a study by Bender.

"According to a study by Bender et al, glycerol rhizotomy (GR) and radiofrequency thermocoagulation with glycerol rhizotomy (RFTC-GR) provide similar pain relief and durability of relief in patients with TN due to multiple sclerosis (TN-MS) and patients with idiopathic TN (ITN). In this study, 68% of the patients with TN-MS who underwent GR were pain free without medications after the procedure, compared with 67% of patients with ITN who underwent GR. In patients who underwent RFTC-GR, 72% of those with TN-MS and 73% of those with ITN were pain free without medications after the procedure. Median time to failure was similar with the 2 procedures (for GR, 20 months in patients with TN-MS and 25 months in patients with ITN; for RFTC-GR, 26 months in the TN-MS population and 21 months in the ITN population."

This result shows a high percentage of success. The number even reached 73%. This shows that the surgeries available today may help and even fully take away the pain caused by our damaged trigeminal nerve.

3) Alternative Therapies

In most cases, when the use of medications and surgery are not entirely successful in achieving the goals of therapy for some individuals, alternative therapies and traditional medicine may be employed to relieve pain. Also, these therapies are used not only for the purpose of pain relief, but to promote general health and well-being of the individual. These alternative therapies and traditional medicine may include the use of acupuncture, acupressure, meditation, Ayurveda, yoga, and the like.

Despite the level of acceptance most of these therapies have gained in different cultures and groups of people, most of them are not fully accepted yet by science. This is due to the fact that most of the time, scientific basis for their use and effectiveness is either lacking, or in worse cases, non-existent. Furthermore, there are numerous methods in which these therapies may be performed and therefore there is no way to ascertain which of these methods would prove to be more effective over the other. Although the choice of having traditional and alternative forms of therapies to cure or treat the presence of trigeminal neuralgia cannot be taken away from the individual suffering from it, he should be properly guided in making the choice. Letting him know about the possible risks and benefits of each therapy may be a good start, as well as examining the manner in which these therapies are performed against his beliefs and values.

Acupuncture

The main principle behind the use of acupuncture in the management of pain in individuals with trigeminal neuralgia is to block the transmission of its sensation from the nerves to the brain. This traditional Chinese medical procedure has been used extensively in Asia for a long time due to its relative effectiveness. In this therapy, long pins or needles are surgically inserted into specific pressure points throughout the body. As the needles or pins are inserted into these pressure points, these are expected to block sensations or impulses traveling in these nerve pathways, thereby reducing the intensity or severity of pain felt by the individual. In some cases, individuals who have undergone this therapy would have several treatments done. These additional treatments are done not only to increase effectiveness but also to promote relaxation and comfort to the individual.

When using acupuncture as a treatment, it is worth to note that those who would want to have it done should look for a person with proper training in using and performing acupuncture. This is because the procedure entails the actual insertion of needles into the nerves and their branches and pathways, and therefore any mistake might cause permanent nerve damage. In most cases, people who are trained to perform acupuncture have certificates to show their proficiency and mastery of this ancient Chinese medical procedure.

Individuals who are afflicted with trigeminal neuralgia undergoing this procedure are usually allowed to relax prior to the treatment. After that, needles and pins are inserted surgically along the trigeminal nerve pathways and its branches along the affected side of the face. In most instances, pain relief is reported immediately after the treatment, although it may be recommended that the needles be left in place for a couple of minutes to a few hours after their insertion to potentiate its effects.

Acupressure

If acupuncture involves the insertion of needles and pins directly into the affected nerves to promote pain relief, the use of acupressure is less invasive than that. In this traditional Chinese medical procedure, pressures are being exerted upon the affected nerves or areas of the body through certain trigger points usually located in the feet. Practitioners of this traditional Chinese medical art commonly use an illustration (of the feet most of the time) that guides them exactly where to exert pressure. This pressure has a specific intensity, and is usually thought to travel from its origin into the affected portion of the body and create a balance in that area. This balance is thought to be what decreases pain sensation in people with trigeminal neuralgia, since an imbalance in the functioning of the trigeminal nerve is what contributes to the pain that is often complained by individuals suffering from it.

One of the advantages of this therapy is that it is non-invasive. This means that there is usually no associated discomfort as the therapy is being performed. This makes it easier to be done at the convenience of the individual. Another advantage of this is that there is a low risk to incur irreversible damage since most of the procedure is performed superficially. Compared with acupuncture, there is almost no risk of increasing or worsening the damage inflicted upon the trigeminal nerve since the pressure points are almost often located elsewhere in the body. A third advantage of this therapy is that it can also be used to promote comfort and general sense of well being of the individual.

There are numerous practitioners of this traditional Chinese medical procedure but it would be worthy to consider the skills and experience of the person that would be chosen to do this. Aside from being certified to have undergone trainings to perform acupressure, it is also important to note the length of time the person has been performing acupressure and where training came from. Mostly, native Chinese practitioners of this ancient form of medicine have learned from family members and the knowledge and skills in acupressure is passed on from one generation to the next.

Chiropractic Medicine

Considered to be an alternative medicine, Chiropractic care is also chosen by those affected with trigeminal neuralgia as a treatment for their condition. The main principle in chiropractice is the identification of the very subtle alignment problems in the spine of the individual. The spinal portion being considered in cases of trigeminal neuralgia is that which is closest to the skull that opens in to the brain stem. This is what is thought to be responsible in rendering management to a number of conditions since the trigeminal nerve is located on this area.

The trigeminal nerve's pathways start from the base of the skull where it exits from its origin in the brainstem and traverses the area along the Atlas bone (the first vertebral bone in the neck area) as it moves to toward the face. This close proximity is responsible for rendering the trigeminal nerve's normal sensory and motor functioning problematic when an alignment defect of the cervical spine happens. Chiropractic procedures performed in individuals with trigeminal neuralgia base on this proximity between the trigeminal nerve and its branches and the state of the cervical spine.

Meditation

Meditation has always been regarded as a way to relax one's mind and create an inner sense of peace and calm. This ancient practice is also used to promote pain relief in individuals who wanted to have therapies that do not require the use of medication and surgeries. There are several forms of meditation being practiced but one of the most effective forms of meditation that can be used in treating the pain associated with trigeminal neuralgia is a mindfulness based meditation practice.

In mindfulness based meditation, the individual is taught about putting all feelings, emotions and sensation to the level of one's awareness. This would allow the individual to understand his pain related to trigeminal neuralgia in terms of its nature and intensity, explore this pain and find ways on how he can deal with it or control it. Since meditation would also require the individual to control his breathing and relax his mind, he would be able to really assess if he is feeling the pain as it is or if his own perceptions affect the level in which pain is felt. This goes on in a continual process until the individual has gained mastery of the practice of meditation and he is able to incorporate the principles of meditation in how he lives his life daily, allowing him to control his pain in the process.

Moreover, the use of meditation is not only limited to decreasing pain perception in individuals with trigeminal neuralgia. It can also be used to manage psychosocial symptoms that the condition brings about. It can be used to manage depression, especially in those who have been afflicted with trigeminal neuralgia for an extended period of time. This is because as the person gains awareness of the nature and severity of his pain and acquired the skills to manage it, he can also go on in focusing on things that are more positive. In doing this, the individual sees more than just the pain and limitations in his activities of daily living that trigeminal neuralgia brings about. He would be able to experience a general sense of well being and be able to carry on his daily tasks independently.

One thing to remember about meditation, however, is that this requires patience and several weeks of practice before a person can do this effortlessly. This is due to the fact that a person would have to be able to focus and not be easily distracted. It is also worth to note that this may not be introduced or suggested to those who are in severe pain and those whose pain levels are not managed well because focus would be almost impossible to achieve when the individual is in severe pain.

Ayurvedic Therapy

Ayurveda is a traditional form of medicine that originated from India. Like other forms of traditional and alternative forms of medicine, Ayurveda aims to provide cure or relief from any symptom the individual feels the natural way. One of the ways to do this in Ayurveda is to determine which symptoms ails the individual the most and targets it directly through the use of medicines, oils, massages or any combination of the three. Ayurvedic treatments are widely used, especially among those who are practicing other forms of alternative medicines, meditation and yoga.

One of the most commonly used Ayurvedic treatment principle in individuals with trigeminal neuralgia is the provision of symptomatic relief and management, decreasing the pain sensation and treating the underlying cause of the problem if it is known. This can be achieved through providing treatments intended to soothe the affected nerve cells and tissues, reducing the appearance of swelling and inflammation. Since the affected trigeminal nerves are likely to be degenerated, there is a possibility that Ayurvedic therapies need to be taken for several weeks or months to note any obvious improvement and be continued still to render complete healing to the damaged trigeminal nerve. If there is the presence of pressure exerted upon the trigeminal nerve by the surrounding vessels like veins or arteries or even the presence of a tumor that is slowly growing, there are also appropriate Ayurvedic medicines to relieve them.

Other than being used to actually treat and provide cure for trigeminal nerve injury and provide permanent natural pain relief to the individual, Ayurveda may also be used to detect the presence of trigeminal neuralgia. This can be done by providing the individual specific doses of Ayurvedic medicines to be taken and a healer trained in this art usually assesses the individual to note for a reduction in the presence of facial pain and the hypersensitivity to stimuli by the trigeminal nerve. When pain is relieved through the use of the administered medication, then it can be deduced that the individual indeed is suffering from trigeminal neuralgia.

Ayurvedic medicines and treatments can also be used, and is therefore needed, in the efforts to improve blood circulation in the affected trigeminal nerve and its branches. This improvement in blood circulation would be helpful in decreasing the pain felt by the individual, allows the person to function independently and optimally, and ensure that nerves have higher chances of healing and recovery. Toxins and other chemical substances in the blood of the individual, which can either trigger an attack of trigeminal neuralgia and worsen it or even prolong it are also treated through Ayurveda. Similar with the management and protocol used for trigeminal neuralgia diagnosis and treatment, the person may need to wait several weeks to several months before noticeable effects occur, and even longer to render cure to the condition. When used properly and conscientiously, Ayurvedic practices and medicines can help tremendously in the management and even the treatment of individuals diagnosed with trigeminal neuralgia.

Traditional or Herbal Medicines

Each culture has their own means of treating certain conditions and pain is one of the most common conditions that people have complained of since the beginning of time. Individuals with trigeminal neuralgia are no exception to this, and traditional medicinal practices have their own treatments for this.

In traditional Chinese herbalism, the presence of trigeminal neuralgia is believed to be caused mainly by the presence of an imbalance in the environment and temperatures (wind, damp and heat). This would mean that the treatments are aimed to address these problems since they believe that managing the underlying cause can greatly enhance efficiency of treatments. Managing these would entail the application of gentian violet into the affected facial area and prescribing the individual with trigeminal neuralgia to take oriental wormwood are thought to be beneficial.

- Folk medicine, however concentrates more on treatment options that are readily available at the home and can be done by the individual diagnosed with trigeminal neuralgia himself. Most of these include the use of oils that can be applied into the affected area or teas, which can be drank to promote pain relief.

- Rubbing either peppermint or clove oils (rubbed inside the mouth) into the affected facial areas are usually recommended as well as rubbing lemons into the face.

- The intake of celery juice or celery tea is thought to decrease the pain.

- Warm cider vinegar compresses are also used to promote relief from pain.

- Aromatherapy can also be done to promote pain relief, enhance blood circulation to the facial area and affected trigeminal nerve branches and to promote relaxation and calmness. Massaging the affected sides of the face with eucalyptus, lavender or chamomile oils can help increase blood circulation to the affected area and promote pain relief while infusing these herbs to the bath can also have the same purpose.

- Application of warm compresses with rosemary oil also increase blood circulation to the affected trigeminal nerve pathways and encourage healing of the injured nerve.

- Mustard and pepper oils, as well as grape seed oils, can also be used in combination for massaging into the affected facial areas.

Blend 1 drop each of mustard and pepper oils in some grapeseed oil and massage into the affected area.

- In the perspective of herbalism, the use of rosemary and lavender infusions as tea and drank by those with trigeminal neuralgia can help relieve severe facial pain. Cayenne-infused oils may also be used for its capacity to promote warmth into the affected facial area. Easing inflammatory process and promotion of pain relief can also be attained though the use of applying a warm chamomile compresses into the affected nerve pathways.

- Homeopathy can also be used to treat the symptoms brought about by trigeminal neuralgia. However, it is important that the use of homeopathic treatments be administered or closely supervised by an individual trained in homeopathic remedies. In this form of alternative therapy, the use of preparations should also be closely followed because wrong constitutions of the preparation may bring about adverse effects. In homeopathy, arsenicum may be used for pain brought about by dry cold temperatures, Lachesis for pain that usually increases in intensity after the individual sleeps and magnesium phosphate is the pain that the person feels decreases in intensity when pressure and heat is applied to the affected area.

- Also, aconite may be used for those who are experiencing symptoms that occur suddenly, most especially after they are exposed to cold temperatures.

- Colocynthis may also be used if the person suffers from pain caused by exposure to cold or damp temperatures.

- The effectiveness of willow barks to remedy pains has been recognized throughout history. It acts like aspirin that is used against headaches, menstrual pain, muscle pain arthritis and diseases of the spine. Early accounts on the use of the bark dated back to Hippocrates' time where people are advised to chew on the bark of the willow tree to relieve muscle pains and headaches and fever. The willow bark is also used for the common flu and even weight loss. These barks contain salicin, an active ingredient also found in aspirins. However, dosage must be proper for over dosage may lead to death. Music legend Ludwig von Beethoven's death is speculated to be caused by extreme dosage of salicin. The willow tree is also composed of plant chemicals polyphenols and flavonoids, which are believed to have antioxidant, antiseptic and immune-boosting powers. Willow barks have different variations including the white willow, the black willow, crack willow and purple willow. All types are used as pain relievers though the most common are the black and white willow tree barks.

- Salicylates, ingredients found in aspirin, are also found in meadowsweet, a plant that grows above the ground. Both the flower and the leaves can be used. Although this plant is more popular to relieve stomach pains, it is also relieves and remedies pains caused by trigeminal neuralgia. It also treats pains in any kind of nerve endings.

- Sweet woodruff helps to fight insomnia, which is a side effect of trigeminal neuralgia. This plant gives off a relaxing and calming feeling to the body, which relieves the stress and tension from people. Another plant that is being used by trigeminal neuralgia patients is the betony. It relieves pains in the face and head. It can be consumed as a tea and after a few weeks of continuous consumption, it will heal facial and head pain.

Biofeedback

Actions such as clapping our hands, raising our hands to smack a high five, waving hello to a friend, kicking and winking are actions that people can control. The rest of our bodily functions such as heart rate, body temperature and blood pressure are involuntary actions created by the central nervous system. Involuntary movements are our body's response to our environment. Incidents like nervousness, excitement and body exertions such as exercise are factors for involuntary movements.

However, science provided a way for people to have a better grasp on their control functions. Biofeedback, a technique used to help the participant gain more control to the usual involuntary mechanisms in the body. People in the medical field use this therapy to treat or merely prevent conditions including chronic pain, high blood pressures, migraines and other sickness involving the brain. The idea of this therapy is that a person can gain more control over involuntary body functions resulting in more control over the person's health, all by harnessing the power of the mind and be aware of the body's movements and changes.

On biofeedback sessions, electrodes, which send signals to the monitor through lights, sounds or images that projects representations of involuntary movement like sweating, heart and breathing rate, blood pressure muscle movements and blood pressure, are attached to the skin.

There are different kinds of biofeedback, but the most common used for patients with trigeminal neuralgia is the neurofeedback or electroencephalography (EEG). The EEG is used to measure brain waves and helps detect seizure disorders including attention deficit hyperactivity disorder (ADHD) and epilepsy. Doctors treating trigeminal neuralgia use this type of biofeedback to help the patient focus on making small and subtle changes in the body. Relaxing certain muscles in the body to reduce pain is the main purpose of the therapy. Biofeedback, specifically neurofeedback, gives the patient the power to use thoughts to control the body most likely to improve debilitating chronic disorders and help with the patient's health condition and physical performance.

Stem Cell Therapy

This type of therapy is still under controversy as to its relative use and effectiveness in treatment of various conditions. However, more and more people are trying stem cell therapy because of the promise of the therapy to return them to their state of health before their diagnosis is made, or in even better shape than that.

In stem cell therapy, fresh stem cells usually harvested from the individual himself, or from other sources are introduced to his body via an injection of myeloid and endothelial progenitor cells. These often young or immature cells are not yet differentiated, meaning they do not have a specific purpose or function yet prior to their introduction. What these cells do after they are introduced to the individual with trigeminal neuralgia is that they go into specific target tissues and start to multiply there. This multiplication or cellular division process results into growth of new nervous system tissues within the affected trigeminal nerve area. These new tissues carry on the normal functioning of the trigeminal nerve, but since they are regenerated tissues, the problem with functioning is either significantly reduced or entirely resolved.

Also, because regeneration is achieved with the introduction of stem cells, other underlying problems within the trigeminal nerve and its branches are also managed such as impairment in the blood circulation and lesions that may have contributed to the occurrence of the trigeminal nerve injury and subsequent diagnosis of trigeminal neuralgia. Moreover, since problem areas are corrected and severely injured or even dead tissues have been regrown, the treatment promises permanent results and continuous improvement as these cells influence the surrounding tissues in their regeneration. This means that there is a very high possibility of a higher level of functioning of the trigeminal nerve can be achieved if the individual opts to go for this treatment. Most of those advocating the use of stem cell therapy also claim that the procedure would be able to bring about noticeable changes, and even pain relief, after a couple of treatments.

However, the use of stem cells, as mentioned earlier is still not widely known or supported by a lot of literatures. Therefore, most physicians are still skeptical to its use and relative efficiency in the treatment of individuals with trigeminal neuralgia. Unlike other treatments that may be classified as either alternative or traditional, stem cell therapies also cost more because it is more complicated to perform compared with other regimens. Despite its promise to allow the individual to achieve pain relief and long term benefits, the risks associated with this relatively new and still controversial treatment would have to be examined.

Chapter 6: Trigeminal Neuralgia and Dental Procedures

Much of medical literature about trigeminal neuralgia never fails to include in their discourses the relationship between the existence of trigeminal neuralgia and dental problems and dental procedures. As several professors from the University Of Florida College Of Dentistry (Gainesville, Florida) and the Parker E. Mahan Facial Pain Center have discussed, there is a relatively significant link between trigeminal neuralgia and dental problems.

Over the years, statistics have shown that most individuals diagnosed with trigeminal neuralgia have had previous experiences of being misdiagnosed with a dental problem. This prompts them to see dentists and get treatments such as tooth extractions and root canal procedures unnecessarily. This problem happens because the nature of the symptoms of trigeminal neuralgia can be triggered during routine dental examinations as well. The usual symptoms of facial pain that is triggered by tapping of the teeth during dental assessments can be interpreted as sign of the dental problem pulpitis. Pulpitis is characterized by the presence of inflammation of the nerve or the pulp of the tooth. When this happens, the individual is usually advised to undergo root canal as treatments of choice. However, not all of those who were positive for tooth pains have trigeminal neuralgia.

1) What Dentists Should Do

An extensive history and assessment should be carried out by the dentist when an individual complaining of facial pain comes in for a checkup. This includes asking very detailed and specific questions about the nature and other factors associated with the pain. Most dentists do tests for the general health of the tooth being complained about by most of their patients through subjecting it to hot or cold compresses and checking for the presence of pain. If either of the two compresses triggers facial pain, then it is likely that the individual has pulpitis. But prior to instituting any form of aggressive therapies or surgical management, it is important that an assessment on a medical standpoint also be made to rule out other causes of facial pain.

In some instances, individuals who were often misdiagnosed to have dental-related facial pains instead of trigeminal neuralgia present with a symptom that occurs as a precursor to it. The individual with this precursor symptom usually complains of pain that is sporadic in nature, and may be described as a stabbing sensation that is typically seen in those with classic trigeminal neuralgia. In others, the pain can also be described as a dull aching sensation that is intermittent in nature. The problem with this precursor symptom is that the pain is not normally associated with the introduction of a stimulus in any specific trigger zone, although certain factors can bring about the attack of pain. These are facial muscle movements associated with talking, chewing, yawning, drinking cold liquids, or even brushing of the teeth. One of the best ways to arrive at a definitive diagnosis is to render the affected area numbed through the use of long acting local anesthesia. If the individual indeed has a dental problem, the pain relief rendered by the anesthesia is short-lived and additional doses might be required to achieve the same effect. However, in individuals who have trigeminal neuralgia, the pain relief brought about by the introduction of anesthesia is long lasting and the relief may even be felt despite the wearing off of the anesthetic agent. When this happens, most individuals are usually given doses of anesthetic agents to provide pain relief for a longer duration of time, spanning a minimum of weeks to years.

2) The Role of Dental Works on Trigeminal Neuralgia Pain

Dental procedures, especially those that are considered to be major works, can either be a positive or negative factor in triggering the pain associated with trigeminal neuralgia. Some major dental procedures can either end the pain, or become its triggering factors in some individuals. This can be attributed also to the failure of some dental procedures to render pain relief to individuals with trigeminal neuralgia. In worse cases, the performances of certain dental procedures are actually linked to the occurrence of break through pain. Breakthrough pain is defined as the presence of severe or excruciating pain in an individual who has pain levels controlled over a prolonged period of time. This pain usually comes on suddenly, with no exact factor triggering it. This makes it hard to manage individuals with trigeminal neuralgia from a dental standpoint because although dental procedures can contribute greatly to the efforts to provide pain relief, it can also trigger the occurrence or worsening of symptoms associated with trigeminal neuralgia. Because of this, dental procedures and assessments are recommended to those with trigeminal neuralgia only when they are of utmost importance. This means that more conservative dental treatments should always be considered and done first if major work-ups and procedures can still be delayed to avoid triggering facial pain.

3) Recommendations for Undergoing Dental Procedures in Individuals with Trigeminal Neuralgia

Although there is the possibility and the need to delay all major dental works to prevent triggering an episode of intense facial pains in those diagnosed with trigeminal neuralgia, there are times that these procedures cannot just be postponed any longer. If it is really necessary for the person to undergo dental work-ups, giving pre-emptive pain relief measures through the use of anesthesia can be done. This is to prevent the development of breakthrough pain from happening while the procedure is being done. The following steps can be taken to ensure that when dental works of the major nature can no longer be delayed, pain can still be prevented and managed.

1. If already diagnosed with trigeminal neuralgia prior to dental works, make sure that there is an order of increased dosage of pain medications from the physician a day or two prior to the treatment.

2. If the application of local anesthetics is indicated, ensure that the dentist would be administering a type of anesthetic with added epinephrine such as Marcaine. Epinephrine just acts to constrict blood vessels, so if this anesthetic is used, the efficiency of pain relief and numbness is affected by its absorption, requiring more doses and multiple shots to attain a desired state of anesthesia. One advantage of Marcaine as an anesthetic agent is that it is long-acting. This means that the need for multiple doses is minimized because the individual stays pain-free for longer periods of time.

3. Ensure that the anesthetic agent is introduced to a nerve site or branch that is considerably far from an identified trigger point to avoid experiencing severe or even breakthrough pain.

4. Pain killers such as codeine and other types of pain medications can also be taken a few hours prior to any procedure to potentiate pain relief rendered by anesthetic agents. This also helps in ensuring that there is a minimum of at least five hours of window period from the pain associated with trigeminal neuralgia. A word of caution, however, ensures that the use of pain killers is prescribed by a physician for safe use.

5. In some individuals who usually get nervous prior to the start of any dental procedure, emotional trauma and triggering of pain sensations related to stress may be reduced through the introduction of sedatives.

4) Adjustments Necessary in Terms of Dental Health

In some individuals who are diagnosed with trigeminal neuralgia, tooth brushing everyday becomes a painful experience, and something that they want to avoid if possible. This can be remedied by having the dentist prescribed an anesthetic that can be applied on the gums to numb the area with severe pain. This preparation is mostly viscous lidocaine solution. If the use of this topical anesthetic is not enough to render the individual pain-free, another preparation can be used in the form of a mouth wash. This solution is an oral antibiotic and can be obtained only with a valid prescription from a licensed dental practitioner. However, this oral antibiotic has the tendency to leave stains on the teeth so it is imperative to ensure that the teeth are thoroughly wiped after each intake so that no residues are left. The intake of fluids that have lukewarm temperature is also encouraged so that the nerves responsible for triggering pain sensation is not stimulated.

These simple measures are helpful in contributing to avoid breakthrough pains and exacerbation of pain related to trigeminal neuralgia. It is essential, however, that the individual gets periodic dental prophylaxis (or teeth cleaning) done so that the risk of plaque and cavity formation is reduced and any dental problems starting to occur are controlled as soon as possible.

Chapter 7: Adapting to the Problem of Trigeminal Neuralgia

Most people with trigeminal neuralgia suffer from the condition for a considerable amount of time due to late diagnosis of the problem, wrong diagnosis or even wrong treatment regimens instituted. For those who were able to get diagnosed early, there is a need to adapt to the condition because of the impairment in several areas of functioning of the affected trigeminal nerve pathways. It is also important that these changes and adaption to the condition be started as early as possible to help the individual deal not only with the pain which is the main symptom of trigeminal neuralgia, but also with the other problems related with the disease. Furthermore, the family of the individual also need to help them in adapting to the condition, also decreasing the risk of depression to occur and other related psychosocial problems.

1) Lifestyle Changes

Trigeminal neuralgia and its symptoms may progress over time and the severity of symptoms and degree of suffering that the person experiences depend on the adjustment he has to make. These adjustments have to be made every day and have to be adapted to not only by the person but also their family as well. Since the attacks of trigeminal neuralgia can be influenced by certain triggers such as the weather, noise and even lighting conditions, there is a need for the individual to modify their daily activities to ensure that attacks are not triggered by extremes in these factors. Moreover, because the environment cannot be modified, a general plan for adapting to it in an effort to decrease pain perception should be in place.

As mentioned in the previous chapters of this book, trigeminal neuralgia can also be caused by a problem in blood supply and circulation to the affected trigeminal nerve and its branches. Lifestyle habits, such as cigarette smoking and alcohol intake should be minimized, if not entirely avoided to decrease the attacks and progression of pain. This is because cigarette smoke is known to cause the release of adrenalin from the adrenal glands. Adrenalin, when it is in high levels of concentration on the blood stream causes constriction of blood vessels, affecting the efficiency of blood circulation. Alcohol, on the other hand, has an oxidizing effect to the cells and tissues of the body. This can increase the progression of damage to the trigeminal nerve tissue, causing the injury to extend, further deteriorating the myelin sheath that covers it and contributing to the pain.

Adapting to the problem is a long-term process and would require not just commitment from the individual but also patience, since it would not be easy for anyone to modify the things they got used to and deal with the pain at the same time. The family can also help in instituting lifestyle changes necessary through encouraging the person on his way to adaptation, and at the same time modifying their activity plans and lifestyle patterns as well not just to fit to those being adhered to by the individual but also in an effort to minimize the risk and possibility of developing trigeminal neuralgia themselves.

2) Dietary Changes

Trigeminal neuralgia affects not only the sensory functioning of the affected trigeminal nerve and its branches, but also their motor function as well. Apart from the pain that is one of the most common symptoms complained about by almost all of those who have it, there are also problems with the motor functioning of the nerve, affecting the movements of the muscles along the trigeminal nerve branches and pathways that innervate them. This can lead to problems with opening the mouth, chewing and even swallowing. Moreover, because of the presence of pain, most of those diagnosed with the problem have decreased nutritional intake, further affecting their bodies' capacity to heal and regenerate the affected trigeminal nerve or recover from any therapeutic procedures performed to alleviate the problem.

Dietary modifications are essential to be made, not only to help adaptation to the problem but also to ensure general well being of the affected individual. These modifications may be introduced slowly over time to ensure that the person would adhere to them, since any sudden change might bring about stress, and complicate the already painful experience associated with the diagnosis of trigeminal neuralgia.

1. *Soft foods*. To ease the need for more forceful or longer chewing that is needed to break down food and decrease the risk of triggering an attack of facial muscle pain, the individual can be started on a diet consisted of foods with softer consistencies. These foods can still contain and involve those that the person has preference to, but just have to be prepared so they are softer. For example, the person likes potatoes, instead of going for fries, which would entail chewing longer; mashed potatoes can be prepared instead.

2. *Increased fluids*. Increasing fluids in the diet of the individual would serve to hydrate him, contribute to enhancing blood circulation and general well being. In the individual with trigeminal neuralgia, increasing the intake of fluids can facilitate

easier chewing and eventual swallowing of foods and increasing the nutritional intake in those who are diagnosed with trigeminal neuralgia.

3. *Increase intake of protein rich foods.* Protein is not only helpful in ensuring tissue repair and regeneration, but it also contains essential B-vitamins that can help maintain and improve the condition of nervous system tissues. This can help enhance the regeneration of the myelin sheath that is lost on the trigeminal nerve and its branches in individuals affected with trigeminal neuralgia, especially if this is done as a part of a treatment regimen. In many cases, Vitamin B supplementation is also one of the lines of treatment as a nerve tonic along with other essential micro-nutrient supplementation, known as Vitamin therapy.

4. *Ensure adequate caloric intake.* Because of the presence of intense facial pains and the possibility of these pains being triggered by activities related to eating such as opening the mouth, chewing and swallowing, people who are suffering from trigeminal neuralgia may have poor caloric intake. This can be remedied through offering small portions of food several times a day to meet daily needs and ensure that the patient is getting the right amount of nutrients needed for faster recovery. Moreover, since other dietary modifications can affect the appetite of the individual, there is also a need to include them in meal planning so that the preference they have for foods should be taken into consideration. The diet that needs to be provided to the individual should focus and revolve around the foods that he or she prefers the most and modifying their preparation to encourage adequate intake.

5. *Avoid taking beverages that are either too hot or too cold.* Extremes in temperatures are one of the pointed causes of pain attacks associated with trigeminal neuralgia. Because the injured

trigeminal nerve is more sensitive to stimuli as compared to a healthy one, the hypersensitivity of the nerve can bring about an episode of pain when exposed to overly hot or cold beverages. It is best recommended that individuals who are suffering from trigeminal neuralgia take beverages at room temperature. In instances where intake of hot beverages such as teas and coffee cannot be avoided, having these in less extreme temperatures can help.

6. *Consider limiting the intake of caffeinated beverages.* In some research studies conducted, caffeinated beverages such as teas and coffee have been found to exert the same effects that cigarette smoking has over the cells and the circulation. They are also related to cause constriction of the blood vessels, which can contribute to injuring the trigeminal nerve and causing increased pain sensations.

7. *Avoid or minimize intake of foods that are associated with increased inflammatory response.* Foods such as those that are high in fat, preservatives, sodium and added sugars in it are linked to increase the development in inflammation in the cells of the body. These foods should be avoided as much as possible so as to decrease the inflammation of the trigeminal nerve, and thereby the symptoms associated with its injury. Moreover, these foods are also those that are advocated in other health conditions such as heart diseases, so eliminating or limiting them from the diet is beneficial not only to address the presence of trigeminal nerve injury but also in preventing other health conditions too.

8. *Work with the doctor and a nutritionist in planning the diet.* There are numerous dietary fads out there about trigeminal neuralgia that can be followed by the individual just to ensure that their pain would be relieved. Since some of these fads are not necessarily supported by research findings and may even prove to

be harmful to the individual, consulting a physician and nutritionist in planning the diet should be considered. This is to ensure that the adjustments to the food intake regarding its types is medically sanctioned and found not to contribute negatively to the condition.

9. *Consider the need to take dietary supplements.* This is to enhance the nutritional status and over-all health and well being of the individual. Most of the therapies involving dietary changes would include the need to take more vitamins and minerals to maintain general health and well being especially when the quality and quantity of food intake is affected by the presence of facial pain. One thing to note, however, is that when dietary supplements are taken, it should be cleared with the doctor first to ensure that the right dosage is taken and that the health of the individuals suffering from trigeminal neuralgia is not compromised.

10. *Plan meals around schedules that allow adequate rest for facial muscles innervated by the facial nerves.* This ensures that the affected areas of the face are not overly stressed or taxed because of meals. Having the individual with trigeminal neuralgia take in small portions of food every 2 to 3 hours throughout the day would help. Resting the affected facial portions might contribute positively to decreasing episodes of pain.

There may be more dietary management, adjustment and considerations that can be done to address the need of individuals with trigeminal neuralgia not only to limit the frequency and severity of the attacks but also to ensure adequate nutritional intake. What is important to remember and note is that there will always be fads that would arise every now and then that would claim to be able to bring about pain relief, and sometimes even a cure without the use of medicines and surgical management and other forms of therapies. The individual, their family and of course the health care professionals who are related to his care should work hand-in-hand to address these issues related to diet so that the person does not fall a victim to these fads.

3) Therapies

In other cases, consulting with a physical or occupational therapist can also be done to help deal with the functional deficiencies that the presence of trigeminal nerve injury and the fear of causing or experiencing pain can bring about. Physical therapy may be availed by the individual increasing the strength of facial muscles that have become weak or paralyzed because of the condition, as its complication, or as a side effect of a treatment regimen. This is highly important because the very basic function of opening and closing the mouth associated with speaking, taking in food and chewing would not be efficiently carried out without adequate muscle strength of the face. Also, the movements associated with the massages and other physical therapy regimen in the affected facial muscle can enhance blood circulation, increase the oxygen and nutrient delivery to the affected trigeminal nerve and its branches, and in the end may contribute to tissue regeneration and growth. Also, the massage can help in relieving facial muscle spasms and enhance other pain relief measures.

Occupational therapy, on the other hand, can be done to help the individual to adapt to the difficulty that goes with the presence of trigeminal nerve injury and facial pain. With occupational therapy, ways of increasing the efficiency of facial muscle movements without adding strain or pressure and causing pain are usually taught to the individual. These seemingly easy modifications taught on occupational therapy are highly important in ensuring that the individual would be able to successfully carry out tasks related to the functioning of the facial muscles that are integral with daily life. Moreover, occupational therapy can also help in ensuring that despite the presence of functional limitations associated with trigeminal neuralgia, the individual suffering from it can still maintain his independence in the activities of daily living.

When either physical or occupational therapy is employed as part of the management during the acute phases of trigeminal neuralgia or a part of a longer course of regimen designed to help the person adjust to the changes that the condition can bring about in his life, full cooperation of the individual is important. This can be obtained through clearly explaining to the person the need for these therapies and how it can help them deal with the problems brought about by trigeminal neuralgia.

4) Dealing with Psychosocial Problems

Feelings of isolation and depression as well as powerlessness and hopelessness are some of the most common psychosocial conditions that can occur when a person is diagnosed with trigeminal neuralgia. These problems occur due to a singular factor and that is the severe pain that the person feels with trigeminal neuralgia. However, in some cases the presence of depression may occur even prior to being diagnosed with the problem because of the long periods of time that the person has dealing with his pain alone and the fact that more often than not, trigeminal neuralgia is either misdiagnosed or dismissed as hypochondriasis. This further isolates the individual not only from health care professionals who are expected to care for them, but also from the rest of the society due to the fear of being stereotyped as having a psychological problem. Moreover, the feelings of hopelessness and powerlessness occur when the person is left to deal with his pain and that several treatments have proved to be ineffective in managing his pain. These psychosocial problems are what put the individual at high risk to contemplate on suicide in the hopes of ending their suffering and ease their perceived burden to their families.

Addressing these psychosocial problems is also as important as the other forms of treatments since the perception of pain can either be masked by these problems or amplified by it. The individual needs to be properly examined for the presence of these problems and once determined, these have to be addressed as soon as possible. In most cases, the best way to determine the presence of psychosocial problems is through the carrying out of conversations with the individual to note for their feeling tone and emotional status. These would have to be made known to the person, since some psychosocial problems may be covert and existing even without the knowledge of the person. When the presence of these problems is determined, some of the following things are done to address them and prevent them from giving birth to other more complicated problems.

1. *Establishing a trusting relationship with the individual.* This is necessary to elicit vital information about the presence of any psychosocial problems. This should be genuine since the person who is suffering from pain related to trigeminal neuralgia has the tendency to be overly sensitive and emotionally vulnerable. Also, mutual trust is necessary to be set between the individual suffering from trigeminal neuralgia and his family and those who are tasked with the responsibility of addressing his psychosocial needs.

2. *Allowing the individual to talk about his feelings.* This step not only enhances the examination of the person to the presence of

psychosocial problems, it can also help in decreasing the severity of these problems and in the long run help in the resolution of these. This is because as the individual talks about how he is feeling more emotionally, its impact and severity is relieved, knowing more people are knowledgeable about what he going through.

3. *Showing understanding.* One of the most common reasons why emotional and other psychosocial problems increase in their severity is when the person feels no one understands what he is going through. Most people diagnosed with trigeminal neuralgia are led to thinking suicidal thoughts based on this same premise, so understanding is important so that their fears and worries are allayed.

4. *Do not isolate the person.* Trigeminal neuralgia may cause severe pain and limitations in the functional capacity of the individual, but isolation from other people is not the best way to allow the person to rest in all situations. Isolating actually decreases the interaction of the person with others, and allows him more time to concentrate on any possible discomforts he may be feeling. This isolation also tends to amplify the pain and the feeling that he is left alone in dealing with it.

5. *Assure support.* Aside from understanding that the person feels pain, is in pain or fears that pain may occur, there is also the need for the person to be assured that he is not alone. This assurance must also include that there is support for the person psychosocially if he needs it and that there are people willing to help him.

6. *Consider support groups.* Sometimes, one of the best ways to deal with any condition, especially that which is chronic in nature is to encourage the individual to adapt with it. Adaptation would

be easier for the person to do if the encouragement and support comes not only from his family and loved ones but also from those who are experiencing the same problems that he has but are able to deal with it successfully. Support groups about trigeminal neuralgia are present to help people deal with trigeminal neuralgia and are offering this help to almost anyone who needs it. Advantages of having a support group also extend to the family, enabling them to cope with the situation together with the individual affected with trigeminal neuralgia.

5) General Tips to Alleviate Pain

Since pain is the most frequently complained of symptom of trigeminal neuralgia and the symptom can also bring about the presence of other problems, it is important for individuals diagnosed with trigeminal neuralgia to be able to deal with pain independently when and where they need it the most. The tips listed below are aimed at meeting that end.

1. *Provide the person a place where they would feel comfortable and safe to be in.* as mentioned in the previous sections, seclusion is not a good choice for people who are suffering from severe chronic pain associated with trigeminal neuralgia. Interaction with other people should be encouraged, if not physically then by any other means as long as safety of the individual is maintained as well as his level of comfort.

2. *Interact.* Having an interaction with people who suffer is a good source of support as well as instrumental in contributing to feeling better emotionally. This is because the people interacting can relate to what each other is going through.

3. *Encourage consultations or examinations with good neurosurgeons or neurologists who are experienced in handling trigeminal neuralgia cases.* One of the most comforting things to know about doctors that people affected with trigeminal neuralgia can ever know is that they are in good hands. Knowing how many people the doctor has successfully treated of the condition or the number of uneventful surgeries he has performed. Also, one of the ways to ensure that the doctor the person would be consulting with is to seek referrals from people who have been treated by these professionals. Moreover, there are numerous ways to find information about doctors who are good at managing pain for individuals with trigeminal neuralgia, such as the Internet.

4. *Be involved in the diagnosis and treatment.* One of the reasons most people with trigeminal neuralgia are misdiagnosed is because they are not involved in how the condition is diagnosed, affecting its treatment. Providing accurate information about the pain and other symptoms can be a good step toward this. Also, the individual should be encouraged to ask about usual diagnostic tests such as MRIs or treatment options like a microvascular decompression surgery.

5. *Keep a diary about the complaints.* In most instances, when severe pain attacks the individual, recalling information is not entirely possible. This can be remedied by having a journal or a diary about the symptoms, the manner in which they occur and factors that either trigger an attack or contribute to relief can help in chronicling about the history of the pain associated with the condition. Moreover, treatments and other aids rendered should be included on this, as well as therapies instituted and how these acted to provide pain relief.

6. *Maintain adequate nutritional intake.* The quality of nutrition and not the quality of intake is highly essential to facilitating

tissue regeneration and growth. Increasing intake of essential vitamins and minerals such as Magnesium (usually on a dose of 400 mg per day), Vitamin B complexes and other nutrients is encouraged. Moreover, a diet that is low in fat, but high in fiber and fruits and vegetables should be advocated.

7. *Consider the use of technology called the Alpha-Stim.* This technology is designed to train the affected trigeminal nerves to assume normal functioning again. It can be used as an adjunct therapy together with either physical or occupational therapy and can produce favorable results over a minimum of three weeks. Despite the high costs of acquiring this equipment, the individual should know that this can be covered by a majority of insurance companies because this is approved by the FDA and other agencies in other territories. There are a lot of sources of information about this equipment that can be found in the Internet if the use of Alpha Stim is considered.

8. *Remind the individual about the possible triggers that can cause attacks of intense pains.* Most of these triggers include over stimulation of the affected facial areas such as hugging, breezes or even kissing. When the triggers to the occurrence of pain are recognized, the individual can subsequently make actions to avoid these. Examples of these include wearing scarves on over the affected side of the face with extreme weather conditions, informing family members in which side of the face is affected and even keeping first aid materials with them when they go out of the house or when the weather conditions are known to trigger a painful episode.

9. *If Botox treatments are considered, the opinion of a licensed physician should be obtained.* Botox, or botolinium toxin injections, are mostly used for aesthetic purposes of relieving wrinkles and marks associated with aging. Because of its potential

to render the affected areas paralyzed, the opinion of a doctor should be sought and not a cosmetologist or aesthetician.

10. *Address the pain before it even starts.* Most individuals who report that medications do not effectively manage the pain that they feel have the mistake of not taking their medications at the onset of pain. Most doctors prescribe medications to be taken until the next appointment, so it is wise to keep pain medications with the individual always.

11. Consider the use of ice packs or warm compresses. Another source of pain in individuals with trigeminal neuralgia is the presence of muscle spasms when the trigeminal nerve is irritated. The use of ice packs or warm compresses can help address these problems. Ice packs can be applied intermittently over the painful side of the face during an acute attack to reduce the pain while applying warm compresses can provide comfort and ease muscle spasms.

12. *Relax the muscles of the neck.* Problems with neck alignment can also lead to increasing the intensity of the pain experienced by people with trigeminal neuralgia. Aligning the neck can do wonders in decreasing pain sensations and can be achieved through the use of a towel rolled up and placed behind the neck instead of using pillows

13. *Try diversionary pain relief measures.* The individual suffering from trigeminal neuralgia should be encouraged to explore other measures to provide pain relief, such as the use of music, reading, watching television programs and others. The goal here is to guide the individual's attention away from the nature and severity of the pain and into more productive and positive things.

14. *Explore the use of non-pharmacologic, traditional methods of managing pain.* Breathing exercises, meditation and even yoga can also help in reducing the perception of pain associated with trigeminal neuralgia.

15. *Learn more about the condition.* One of the reasons why the pain often felt by the individual is intensified is the presence of lack of knowledge about it. Finding out information about the cause of the condition and how attacks of severe pain can be triggered would help in preventing the occurrence of attacks. Also, the individual should ask his dentist about the risks of getting a root canal procedure if he considers getting it and how it can affect the symptoms associated with trigeminal neuralgia

Chapter 8: Preventing Trigeminal Neuralgia

As mentioned earlier in this article, the definitive cause of neither the trigeminal neuralgia nor its origin is idiopathic or unknown and speculations about it have yet to be scientifically proved. Though the root of this disease is yet to be discovered, a number of treatments have already been proven to lessen the intensity of painful episodes. There are more than enough options for alleviating the individual's pain should an attack occur. However, there is still no way of preventing the occurrence of the disease, only things to consider in avoiding painful attacks should a person suffer from this illness. Below are some tips to prevent attacks, decrease the number of episodes or reduce the intensity of the pain caused by trigeminal neuralgia.

1. *Have basic knowledge about trigeminal neuralgia.* One of the reasons why the pain often felt by the individual is intensified is due to the presence of misinformation or just lack of knowledge about the illness. Information about the disease can be gained through different means such as looking for a doctor who has had experience dealing with patients also suffering trigeminal neuralgia. A number of books and other printed materials also feature articles about the disorder The World Wide Web and its growing networks are probably the easiest access to such information. Fishing out data and gaining knowledge about the disease is good for early diagnosis of the disorder. If a person who has trigeminal neuralgia grasps the nature of the disease, it would be easier for the individual to manage it. The Clinical Study of Trigeminal Neuralgia also shows how big advantage it is to be aware of what's going on:

"Patients benefit from an explanation of the natural history of the disorder, including the possibility that the syndrome may remit spontaneously for months or even years before they need to consider long-term anticonvulsant medications. For this reason, some may elect to taper off their medication after the initial attack subsides; thus, they should be educated about the importance of being compliant with their medication regimen.

Patients also must be educated about the potential risks of anticonvulsant medications, such as sedation and ataxia, particularly in elderly patients, which may make driving or operating machinery hazardous. These drugs may also pose risks to the liver and the hematologic system. Document the discussion with the patient about these potential risks.

No specific preventative therapy exists. Patients may have a premonitory atypical pain for months; therefore, appropriate recognition of this pre–trigeminal neuralgia syndrome may lead to earlier and more efficient treatment.

Patients should avoid maneuvers that trigger pain. Once the diagnosis is established, advise them that dental extractions do not afford relief, even if pain radiates into the gums.

In patients wishing to undergo a procedure, they should be aware of potential adverse effects, as well as report any altered sensation in the face, especially after a procedure. They should be informed about the potential for anesthesia dolorosa."

2. *Identify your trigger buttons.* Trigeminal neuralgia can cause pain even with the smallest sensations and slightest stimulations on the trigeminal nerve. The individual must be able to pinpoint the trigger button activities that cause the disease to act up and frequently cause unforeseen and harsh pain, thus preventing or

putting these types of activities on a downscale. Triggers vary from person to person.

3. *Take note of the progress of the disease.* Tracking the progress of trigeminal neuralgia in an individual can greatly aid in the anticipation of the attacks, especially if activities and treatments are well noted. A thorough record like a journal of the frequency and escalation of the pain and a list of what triggers each episode is to be recorded and made a reference in planning daily activities. Preventive measures such as avoiding past physical activity which caused pain can be done by the use of records.

4. *Be conscious of your intakes.* Essential activities such as eating or more specifically chewing are the most common kinds of triggers. The exertion in the facial muscles causes pain. It is recommended to decide meals to the situation. One option would be to take in more soft foods as to minimize the chewing process. The individual may also choose to consume foods that do not require chewing. Consuming food and beverages of room temperature is also highly recommended. Also, as discussed earlier, poor dietary choices worsens the effect of trigeminal neuralgia to the body so the individual must ensure to consume a good balanced diet.

5. *Stay indoors on a windy day.* A simple force such as a wind breeze can spark a series of painful jabs on the face. During a windy day, it is best for the individual to stay inside the confines of a house. If going outside in such weather conditions is inevitable, be sure to wrap a scarf high on the face of the individual as to inhibit the direct hit of the wind to the face. Furthermore, always keep in mind to change the direction of the air vents of air conditioning units to avoid being in the direct way of the air flow.

6. *Keep lifestyle in good condition at all times.* As discussed earlier in Chapter 3 about the risk factors of trigeminal neuralgia, there are a lot of modifiable risk factors (things that we have control over) that we can manage on our own. Vices such as cigarette smoking increase our risk in having the disorder. A clean bill in cigarettes and practicing safe sex (to avoid herpes) can lessen the possibility of acquiring the disorder.

7. *Search for Alternatives.* Although having trigeminal neuralgia limits the usual routines in everyday life, finding alternatives to all restrictions will help the individual relieve some physical and emotional stress. The aim of the alternatives is to reduce the exertion on the nerves associated with the disease. An example would be using a warm damp cloth or cotton pads when washing the face area instead of rubbing it with your palms. Tooth brushing is another essential activity that is one of the most common causes of pain. Instead of brushing the teeth, the individual may prefer rinsing the mouth with warm water. A lot of options are available for people suffering from the disease.

8. *Know your limits.* It is always encouraged to never let sickness get the best out of our lives. People suffering from trigeminal neuralgia throughout the duration of the disease would accumulate a number of restrictions and may not able some activities they previously enjoyed. In order to still be functional, be sure to distinguish the limits of the individual's physical activity and secure that all movements are to never go beyond the safe zone. Preventing the attack is always preferable than treating it.

Researches about Trigeminal Neuralgia

A lot of questions are still left unanswered with regards to this rare but not unusual disorder in the body. Up to this day, the cause of this disease is still debatable. There are no valuable evidences that would support theories on how this illness started and developed.

As to why women are more prone to have this condition are yet to be answered. Scientists try to focus on the female hormone estrogen as they look at its role in affecting nerve pain activity. Understanding estrogen activity in the body, especially on the pain nerves, may give the scientists a bigger picture of the mechanism in the brain.

The growing number of people suffering prompted different organizations to do further studies on trigeminal neuralgia. The National Institute of Neurological Disorders and Stroke (NINDS), part of the National Institutes of Health, funded projects that will explore the mechanisms of the brain and body involved with chronic pain. Those researches also wish to discover a permanent remedy for trigeminal neuralgia. These projects also wish to determine possible novel diagnostic methods and treatments.

Other National Institutes of Health researches are being funded by the National Institute of Dental and Craniofacial Research.

Chapter 9: Self help information

After the thorough discussion on the previous chapters about the nature of trigeminal neuralgia, its signs and symptoms, treatments options available and even the lifestyle changes the person affected by it has to do in order to deal with and cope with the condition. In this additional chapter, the price tags attached to each treatment regimen, blogs that can be used as sources of information and even links to support groups are included. This information is included in this book to further help people affected with the condition and their family to be able to make decision-making on treatment options easier, and enhance their knowledge and ability to cope with and deal with trigeminal neuralgia.

The Cost of Treatments

Medicines

One of the most common drugs given for individuals diagnosed with trigeminal neuralgia is carbamazepine, and the use of this medicine is on a long-term basis and is a necessity in pain management. The drug costs an average of $4-$18 US dollars (2.40-10.85 UK Pound) per piece, depending on the dosage and the brand of the medicine. In some instances, individuals who have trigeminal neuralgia may have the option of buying tablets that are twice their required dosage and cut it in half to save money.

Other drugs that are used for treatment cost almost in the same range with the figure mentioned above, but what causes the burden to those diagnosed with the problem is the high costs of the medicines and the long-term treatment necessary. On an average, a person may spend roughly $10,000 US dollars (or 6,000 UK Pounds) for medicines alone to relieve pain.

Surgeries

Surgical treatments are usually advised for those who have been unresponsive to pain medications and other less invasive procedures. The surgical treatments average $7,000-$35,000 US dollars (or 4,215-22,000 UK Pounds), depending on the type of procedure to be done and the average length of recovery that the individual needs after the surgery itself. Also, this figure may be slightly higher, even going up to double the amount, if the condition is complicated or when the affected area is located in the part of the face that is harder to access.

Traditional and Alternative Medical Management

These therapies, as said before, are not entirely advocated by medical professionals but are chosen by people who are suffering from facial pains because of their reported effectiveness in relieving pain and promoting calm to those who are undergoing these procedures. Consultations with acupressure and acupuncture therapists may start at $100 dollars (60 UK Pounds) and the meditation classes range from $1,200 onwards (720 UK Pounds). Aromatherapy oils, candles and other herbs vary in prices, but these are minimal so it will be easier for the person with trigeminal neuralgia and their families to avail of them. The problem lies, however, in the availability of these products and where to get them. Most stores that carry traditional Asian medicine, or herbal stores have the herbs listed on the treatment chapter of this book, as well as other wellness shops.

Stem cell treatments, also considered to be alternative form of therapy is quite expensive, with a price tag ranging from $8,000 (or 4,800 UK Pounds) up to $30,000 (18,000 UK Pounds), depending on where the treatments are done and how long the therapies would last. In this type of treatments, countries such as China, Germany and Switzerland are some of the top destinations. Because of the need to travel and stay in these countries where most therapy centers are located, the costs are sometimes doubled to include the expenses of the individual and his travel companions.

Insurance Coverage and Financial Assistance for Individuals with Trigeminal Neuralgia

Most health care insurance plans and companies cover the treatment costs associated with trigeminal neuralgia, but most of the time; this is limited to the more recognized treatment regimens such as the use of drugs and surgery. The amount of health care insurance coverage for trigeminal neuralgia may either be full or partial only, depending on the premiums paid. There are instances, however, when some individuals with the condition have gone through treatments in which their insurance companies or plans refuse to reimburse them or simply pay for them because it is not included in the plan, especially if the treatment option they went for are considered to be either traditional or alternative. Therefore, it is important for the individual with trigeminal neuralgia and their families to confirm with their health care insurance providers about the coverage before considering any treatments.

In the United States, Federal and State health departments may extend assistance in terms of treatment to those who were afflicted with trigeminal neuralgia under the Medicaid program. This is usually given to individuals who were considered to be indigents and cannot afford any of the treatment options. Moreover, the social security system of the United States can also extend financial assistance to its members who will qualify for disability because of a diagnosis of trigeminal neuralgia. In the UK, assistance for those who want to have treatment but cannot afford it may be coursed through the National Health Services. Moreover, in most countries, there are various groups that are extending financial assistance for individuals afflicted with trigeminal neuralgia. Most of these can be contacted and coordinated with through the help of support groups.

Where to Find Help?

The Internet is teeming with information about trigeminal neuralgia and where to find help for it through listings of blogs and support group web pages and contact details. Most of the blog postings were stories of people who were diagnosed with trigeminal neuralgia. The following websites are the leading support group and blog posting sites for people with trigeminal neuralgia and offering tremendous help for both the individual and his family.

1. *LivingwithTN.org.* This is a support group that aims to help individuals with trigeminal neuralgia and their family to adjust and adopt with their condition. It also contains blog postings of those who have suffered from the disease and have tried a treatment that works for them.

2. *TNA.org.uk.* This support group is based in the UK and is for people who want support and additional knowledge about trigeminal neuralgia and how to deal with it on a daily basis.

3. *Hopkinsmedicine.org.* A hospital-run website that offers help and assistance to those dealing with trigeminal neuralgia.

4. *Mdjunction.com/trigeminal-neuralgia.* Offers information about trigeminal neuralgia, available treatment options and tips for daily living with the condition.

There are other support groups out there that have the same ideas as these listed above. What is important in choosing these support groups is that the individual and his or her family and their queries about the condition and other needs in dealing with it are met. One of the greatest advantages in having support groups is that the person can really talk with people who can relate with their problem, making it easier to deal with.

Chapter 10: Conclusion

The main purpose of this book is to educate the non-medical professionals about the debilitating and oftentimes severely painful condition called trigeminal neuralgia. Over the entire course of this book much information has been presented about the condition and its impact not only on those suffering from it, but also their families and health care providers. Despite the increasing number of individuals who are affected with this dreaded condition, it is saddening to know that there is not enough literature that talks about it. The Internet may have multiple sites offering information about trigeminal neuralgia but most of these sites talk about similar things, with some of the information posted on these sites being entirely the same. In worse cases, there are also sites that appear to be sources of advice and information but mislead the individuals.

Because of the presence of these problems, it is important for the person with trigeminal neuralgia to really devote time and effort into obtaining the types of information that can help them deal with the condition and guide them to make the best choices in terms of treatments. This book has discussed different aspects related to trigeminal neuralgia, its occurrence, treatment options available and how to best adapt to the presence of the problem. The following points were highlighted in the entirety of this book:

1. Trigeminal neuralgia a condition affecting the trigeminal nerve that traverses the face.

2. The trigeminal nerve has both sensory and motor functioning, rendering a problem with it to affect most of the face.

3. Severe, debilitating pain felt by those affected with the condition is the most reported symptom and it is triggered by several factors.

4. The condition is caused by an injury to the trigeminal nerve or any of its branches that is secondary to a compressing tumor over the trigeminal nerve, problems with blood circulation in the tributaries of the nerve and other traumatic conditions that can deplete the myelin sheath which is the protective covering of the nerves, increasing its sensitivity to stimuli. This is the cause of facial pain in most individuals diagnosed with the condition.

5. There are 7 known subtypes of trigeminal neuralgia but the most common of all these subtypes is the classic manifestation that is seen in approximately 85% of all diagnosed with the problem.

6. Females and those over 50 years old are most commonly affected with the condition, although it can also be diagnosed in those as young as childhood years.

7. The presence of trigeminal neuralgia is usually determined through a combination of laboratory testing, reports of pain of the individual and the results of examinations done in the physicians' clinics.

8. There are a lot of those who were suffering from the condition who went to unnecessary prolongation of suffering because of being viewed as hypochondriacs or being misdiagnosed as having dental problems.

9. There is a strong link between the existence of trigeminal neuralgia and the presence of dental problems as well as the performance of some dental procedures. Dental problems can worsen the condition, but dental procedures can either relieve an

individual of the pain associated with the condition or worsen it. Examples of this procedure include root canal therapies and tooth extractions.

10. The condition can be treated in a lot of ways. There is the use of medicines, surgical interventions and even alternative and traditional medical practices, all aiming to address the major symptom of pain and treat the condition if possible.

11. Lifestyle changes have to be instituted by the individual to help them to adjust to trigeminal neuralgia and reduce the frequency of painful attacks. Activity patterns should also be adjusted not only to decrease pain sensation, but to also promote independence.

12. It is important for the individual to ensure that his dietary intake is adequate in terms of quantity and quality as well. Moreover, the increase or decrease of several types of food can help tremendously in pain relief efforts.

13. Depression and other psychosocial problems should also be given attention, since these problems are responsible for the individual to consider the possibility of committing suicide. These problems should not be taken for granted.

14. Adjustment and preparedness are keys to ensuring that the symptoms associated with trigeminal neuralgia can be managed and that pain levels are not going to reach severe intensity.

15. Referral to support groups can prove to be highly beneficial not only to the individual but to his family as well. The presence of a support group can decrease the risk for depression and facilitate better adjustment of the individual to the condition.

One more thing to take special consideration of is the need for early diagnosis of the condition to prevent it from worsening and developing into complications or severely affect the individual's quality of life and independence in their activities of daily living. The family also plays a highly integral role in this road to adjustment and recovery with trigeminal neuralgia so their support, understanding and appreciation cannot be understated.

Published by IMB Publishing 2014

116

Printed in July 2019
by Rotomail Italia S.p.A., Vignate (MI) - Italy